Drugs and the Brain

DRUGS AND THE BRAIN

Solomon H. Snyder

**SCIENTIFIC
AMERICAN
LIBRARY**

An imprint of Scientific American Books, Inc.
New York

This is number 18 of a series.

Library of Congress Cataloging in Publication Data

Snyder, Solomon H., 1938–
   Drugs and the Brain.

   (Scientific American Library; 18)
   Includes bibliographies and index.
   1. Psychotropic drugs.   2. Brain—effect of drugs
on.   I. Title.   II. Series.   [DNLM: 1. Brain—drug
effects.   2. Psychotropic drugs—pharmacodynamics.
QV 77 S675d]
RM315.S58   1986   615'.788   86-6687
ISBN 0-7167-5015-5

Printed in the United States of America

Book design by Malcolm Grear Designers

Scientific American Library
An imprint of Scientific American Books, Inc.
New York

Distributed by W. H. Freeman and Company,
41 Madison Avenue, New York, New York 10010
and 20 Beaumont Street, Oxford OX1 2NQ, England

1 2 3 4 5 6 7 8 9 0   KP   4 3 2 1 0 8 9 8 7 6

To the Blech family—

dear, loyal friends and exemplars

of the creative process

Contents

Preface   ix

1 The Brain and Its Messengers   1

2 Opiates   29

3 Drugs for Schizophrenia   61

4 Mood Modifiers   91

5 Stimulants   121

6 Easing Anxiety   151

7 Enlightenment in a Pill   179

8 Prospects   207

   Recommended Readings   213

   Notes   215

   Sources of Illustrations   217

   Index   221

Preface

The ostensible purpose of this book is to give the reader a general notion of what is presently known about the major psychoactive drugs and how they act upon the brain to influence behavior. In the course of introducing these fascinating facts and ideas, however, I have attempted to present another aspect of pharmacology as well: the dramatic detective story of how scientists have used drugs as probes that yield novel and exciting insights into brain function. Because human use of some of these drugs goes back thousands of years and represents some of the most important developments in the history of medicine, I have also tried to emphasize the ways in which such progress has been achieved and the creativity of the process by which the best, most productive investigators have assembled disparate and seemingly contradictory pieces of information into unexpected scientific and therapeutic syntheses. To give the reader a foretaste of some of the diverse processes that contribute to drug discovery, perhaps I ought to describe how I myself became immersed in the world of psychopharmacology.

Writing a book about drugs and the brain is a natural outgrowth of my interests, aptitudes, and prejudices since teenage years. In college I was far better at writing and philosophy than at science, but like many of my friends, I chose to pursue a premedical major; philosophy is hardly a proper vocation for a nice Jewish boy. Although I did not particularly look forward to medical school, I did see it as a vehicle to gain admission to psychiatric residency training, and that is where I had set my sights. In medical school, I eagerly absorbed everything my books and teachers could tell me about the brain, but I approached the rest of my courses perfunctorily at best. One other subject did catch my fancy, however, and that was pharmacology. I found it incredible that simple chemical molecules could bring about such profound changes in the human body, and I was intrigued by the disparity between how drugs were used and what was actually known about them: drugs have long been the primary means of treating most diseases, yet until recently physicians have had little understanding of how most pharmacological agents exerted their therapeutic effects. Needless to say, any drug that affected the brain struck me as being especially interesting.

Considering these personal predilections, it was a most fortunate accident that I should find myself, after internship, fulfilling my military obligation at the National Institutes of Health in Bethesda, Maryland, in the laboratory of Julius Axelrod, perhaps the world's most distinguished investigator of how drugs alter the molecular machinery of the brain. Two years with Axelrod taught me that the process of scientific discovery can be as creative as the act of composing a novel or a symphony. The only difference is that scientists must attempt to test their novel conceptions to see whether or not the new ideas provide accurate descriptions of nature.

In 1965 I moved from the National Institutes of Health to Johns Hopkins University Medical School for psychiatric training, and I have remained there on the faculty ever since. Paul Talalay, then chairman of the pharmacology department, provided me with an operational laboratory while I was still in psychiatric training and continued to foster my professional growth over many years. Joel Elkes, chairman of the psychiatry department, greatly facilitated my somewhat unconventional training in psychiatry, permitting me to skip routine clinical chores and thus allowing me ample time for research. My life still centers on the laboratory, where, in close concert with successive generations of talented medical, predoctoral, and postdoctoral students, I attempt to understand how drugs act in the brain. I owe an enormous debt to these students, with whom I am privileged to engage in daily intellectual duels as we explore what a given experiment might mean and where we should take it next.

In retrospect, it seems that my personal forays in creative innovation began with my studies of the classical guitar, when I was thirteen years old. My teacher, Sophocles Papas (who died during the writing of this preface, at age 92), taught me the intense focus of attention required to achieve new insights, whether in interpreting music or in understanding how a drug works. I learned the frustrations inherent in mastering a piece of music and later was not surprised to encounter similar obstacles in the process of obtaining a desired experimental result. I learned also the transcendent joy to be found in successfully apprehending a new and unprecedented idea. Experience has shown me that this applies to music and science alike.

Solomon H. Snyder
Baltimore, Maryland

Drugs and the Brain

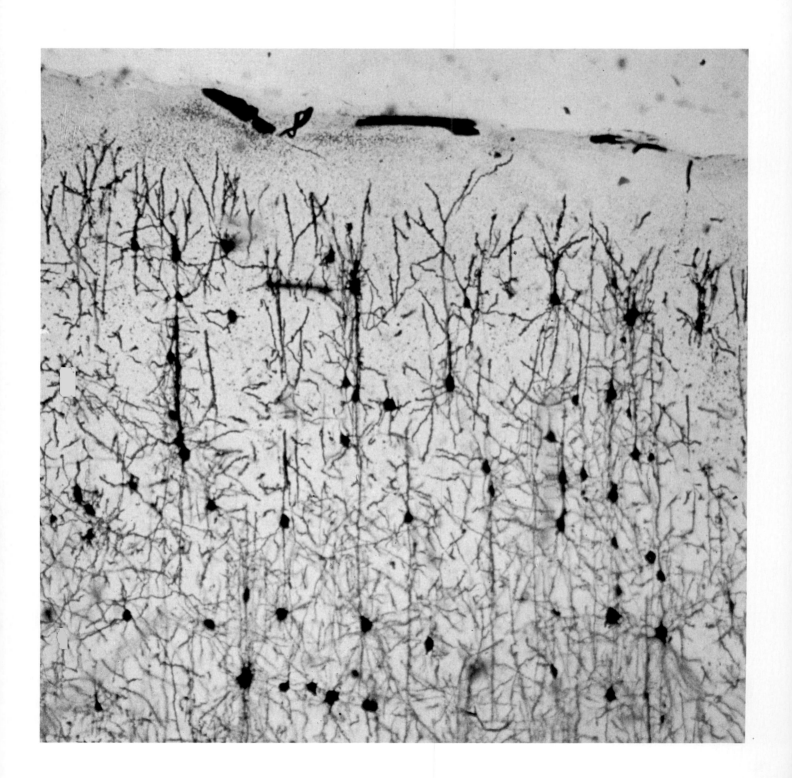

1 | The Brain and Its Messengers

Of all the momentous revolutions of twentieth-century science, two hold particular promise for bringing the mystery of human consciousness into the realm of human understanding. One of these revolutions is the development of new groups of drugs that produce extraordinary effects upon the mind; the other is the explosion in our understanding—at the cellular and molecular levels—of just how the human brain works.

These two fields of inquiry are intimately related. Drugs that affect the brain in novel and unexpected ways reveal hitherto unsuspected facets of brain organization and function. An example is the introduction in 1960 of benzodiazepine drugs, such as the widely used Valium, for the treatment of anxiety. Early in the twentieth century, barbiturates were used to quiet down agitated mental functions; in higher doses, they put the user to sleep—an inconvenient, often dangerous, but presumedly inevitable aspect of any tranquilizing drug activity. The development of benzodiazepine drugs was a startling breakthrough: they were able to calm anxiety without inducing the marked sleepiness brought on by barbiturates. This unique therapeutic utility of the benzodiazepines raises important questions about brain function. The fact that they relieve anxiety without causing much sedation suggests that the alertness system of the brain is different from the anxiety system. Barbiturates and benzodiazepines have provided chemical probes that scientists can use to distinguish between these two functions so as to study them separately.

Drugs differentiate "alertness system" from the "anxiety system"

In the following pages, we will explore the contributions to brain research of several groups of psychoactive drugs, that is, drugs that affect the mind. Some of these drugs are pharmacologically important because of their therapeutic benefits. The antischizophrenic, or neuroleptic, drugs, for example, are widely held to be the most significant drugs in the history of psychiatry. Their use has liberated many schizophrenics from what would otherwise have been a life of confinement in mental institutions. Another group, the antidepressant

Facing page The complex network of neurons that is the human brain regulates all the conscious and unconscious activities that sustain and motivate our lives.

I

A sagittal slice of the human brain.

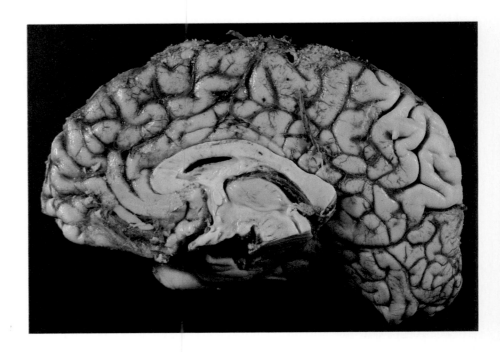

The major classes of psychoactive drugs

Drug class	Examples
Opiates	Morphine Heroine
Neuroleptics (antischizo- phrenics)	Chlorpromazine Haloperidol
Stimulants	Amphetamine Cocaine
Antianxiety agents	Diazepam Chlordiazepoxide
Antidepressants	Amitriptyline Imipramine
Psychedelics	LSD Mescaline
Sedative-hypnotics	Phenobarbital Chloral hydrate

drugs, have successfully aborted long-lasting, excruciatingly painful depressions that, earlier, would all too often have ended in suicide. Finally, antianxiety drugs have freed millions of patients from the affliction of constant, debilitating apprehension.

Others of the drugs we will examine are more often used for recreation than for therapy and are remarkable for the ways in which they have been abused by so many people who, for as yet unfathomed reasons, become slaves to these chemical entities. For thousands of years, opium and morphine, products of the poppy seed, have been used to control pain and to induce euphoria, but only in the last two hundred years has their addictive potential been recognized; their analogue heroin, introduced in the twentieth century, accelerated and accentuated the major opiate effects—the analgesia, the rush of happiness, and the process of addiction. Psychedelic drugs, such as LSD and mescaline, give rise to awesome and extraordinary mental changes in which perceptions are so altered from normal human experience, they cannot readily be described. Cocaine and other stimulant drugs inflate the user's mood so that he or she feels all-powerful and exuberantly fearless.

Pharmacologists, the scientists who attempt to discover the mechanisms whereby drugs exert their effects, have been striving for decades to explain how these drugs act. Within the past twenty years, neuroscientists, the scientists whose primary interest is brain function, have come to realize that psychoactive drugs are powerful tools for unraveling the intricacies of information processing in the brain. The use of these drugs in brain research has already brought about some of the most important recent advances in the neurosciences; and once researchers have discovered, at a molecular level, how these drugs act in the brain to bring about such striking changes in mental processes, they might find it possible to design new therapeutic agents that are far more potent, more efficient, and safer than the ones available now. This reciprocal interaction between drug development for therapeutic purposes and the use of drugs to understand the brain has been largely responsible for an explosion in brain research that began in the 1950s and continues today.

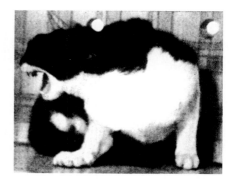

An animal behavior experiment in the laboratory. Electrical stimulation of an area of the hypothalamus causes an aggressive reaction in the cat.

The strategy for using drugs to probe the brain is fairly straightforward. Let us say that a researcher wishes to understand events in the brain that give rise to the subjective feeling of joy. Laboratory researchers often scrutinize the behavior of animals in order to elucidate the general mechanisms by which the human brain functions, but when the subject of inquiry is an emotion, this approach has obvious limitations. Although cats purr and dogs wag their tails, it is unclear whether any animal feels the same emotions in the same way as a human being. Nevertheless, a drug known to produce a feeling of joyfulness in humans can be administered to a laboratory animal, such as a rat, and the nature of the biochemical alterations selectively elicited by that drug can be ascertained. Enough information can be gleaned from observing the changes in the biochemistry of the rat's brain to construct a hypothesis about what happens in the human brain to create a feeling of joy. This description is an oversimplification, and we certainly do not know in detail how the brain regulates joyfulness, but the general strategy has been effective in clarifying many questions about brain function. However, before discussing specific drugs and how scientists have used them to study the chemistry of thinking and feeling, we should briefly survey some basic principles that govern communication between cells in the brain.

Brain Cells

All the psychoactive drugs exert their principal effects upon individual cells in the brain—specifically, upon the points of connection between certain brain cells in certain parts of the brain. Two major cell types account for the bulk of the brain matter: these are the neurons, thought to be the principal information carriers, and the glia, their supporting cells. When a properly stained sample of brain tissue is examined under the light microscope, glia and neurons can be readily distinguished. Most neurons have a long wirelike process that enables them to communicate with other neurons; such processes are lacking in most glial cells.

Although glia comprise about 85 percent of all the cells in the brain, scientists are not certain of their exact functions. In embryos and infants, neurons migrate to assume what will be their adult locations. How this occurs is not yet

Neurons & Glia - brain cells

3

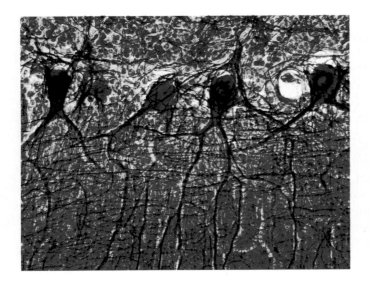 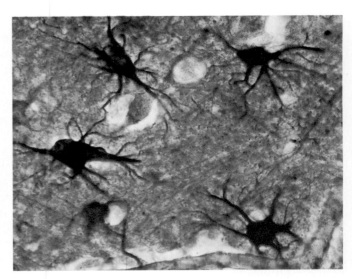

Left Neurons of the human brain. Cell bodies, axons, and dendrites can be distinguished. *Right* Astrocytes, one type of glial cell, multiplied 1000 times.

Axons

Pyramidal Cells - Large neurons

Dendrites

Facing page Neurons can make various types of synaptic connections. Variations include axon with cell body, axon with axon, and axon with dendrite (the "classic" synapse).

understood in detail, but there is strong evidence that glial cells commonly act as guideposts for the migrating neurons. Glia also provide metabolic support to neurons, drawing off neuronal waste products by means of pumplike systems that suck up excess metabolic materials. Some scientists think that in addition glia play a direct role in information processing, but this is a matter of some controversy.

The most remarkable property of the neuron is its ability to transmit information from one place to another more or less distant location. All thinking and feeling is a consequence of the ten billion or more neurons in the brain "talking" to each other. They are uniquely structured for this function. Like all cells in the body, neurons have a nucleus and surrounding cytoplasm, but neurons differ from other cells in that they possess the aforementioned distinctive cellular extensions, called axons, that project information to other, sometimes distant cells. Axons can be extremely long; the large neurons known as pyramidal cells, located in the cerebral cortex, can extend their axons all the way down to the lower part of the spinal cord, a distance of 4 feet in humans and 15 feet in giraffes. The axon's termination, the nerve ending, may divide into as many as ten thousand or more branches, each of which can make contact with a different receiving neuron, thus providing a great diversity of neuronal interconnections.

Nerve endings make contact with other neurons either directly on their cell bodies or, more frequently, on another kind of nerve-cell extension known as the dendrite. Up to ten thousand or more dendrites sprout from a typical neuronal cell, and each dendrite can receive the input of numerous neurons. If we consider the multiplicity of message-receiving dendrites on each neuron, the

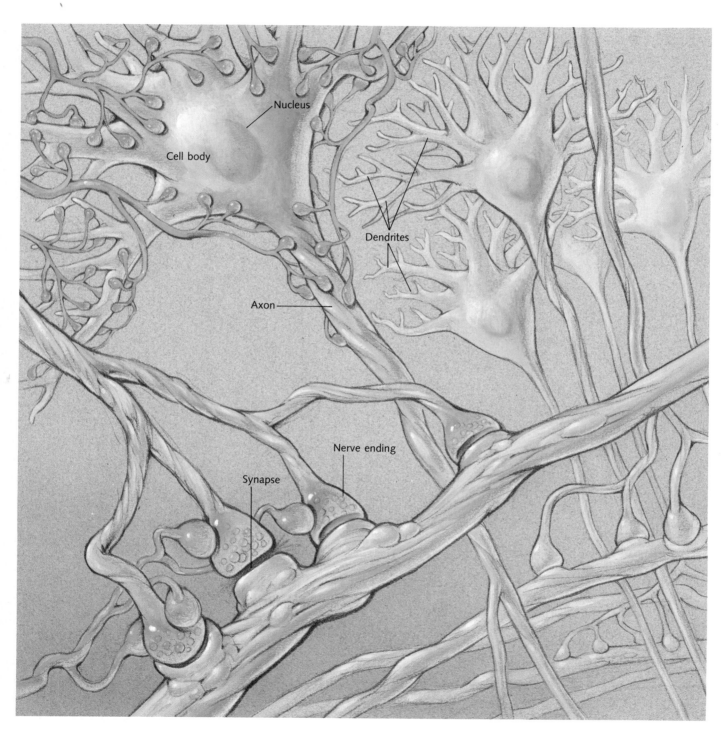

Nucleus

Cell body

Dendrites

Axon

Nerve ending

Synapse

Different types of glial cells. Astrocytes are thought to carry nutritive substances from the blood vessels to the neurons and also to remove potassium and released neurotransmitters from the extracellular space. Oligodendrocytes fabricate the myelin sheath that surrounds and insulates some neurons. Microglia scavenge debris from dead cells. Ependyma line the brain ventricles and regulate the passage of chemicals between the ventricular fluid and the brain substance.

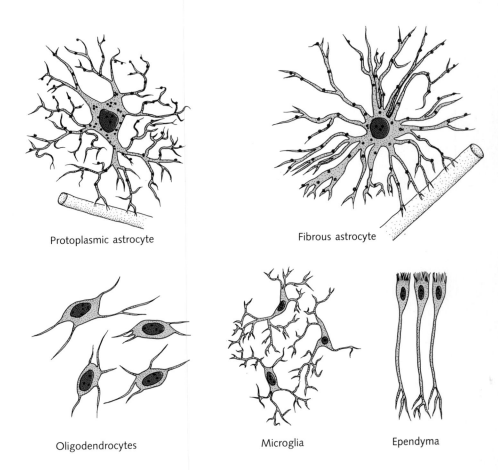

Protoplasmic astrocyte　　　　　　Fibrous astrocyte

Oligodendrocytes　　　　Microglia　　　　Ependyma

thousands of message-distributing branches at the end of each axon, and the billions of neurons in the brain, we quickly grasp that the brain can process a vast array of data.

In the standard depiction of nerve activity, illustrated on the facing page, an impulse arises in the dendrite or cell body and then travels down the length of the axon by a process that is predominately electrochemical in character. The interior of a resting neuron is electrically negative with respect to its exterior, but when a neuron is excited, the electrical potential across the cell membrane is abolished, and the cell's interior may even develop a weak positive charge. Before excitation, the concentration of sodium ions, which carry a positive charge, is normally 25 to 50 times higher outside than inside the axon, but the change in charge across the membrane promotes the entry of sodium ions into the cell. A sudden rush of sodium into the interior at one location on the axon initiates a change in electrical properties at an adjacent location, which causes an inrush of sodium there and propagates the wave of electrochemical activity

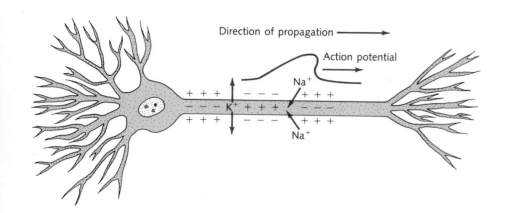

Direction of propagation ⟶

Action potential

In the standard depiction of nerve impulse propagation, the impulse begins in the cell body and travels down the axon toward the nerve endings. As it travels along the axon, the impulse reduces the voltage difference between the interior and exterior of the cell. This allows a local inflow of sodium (Na^+), the event that propagates the impulse. It is followed by an outflow of potassium ions (K^+), which returns the membrane potential to its resting state, ready for the arrival of a new impulse.

that continues down the entire length of the axon. When this occurs, the cell is said to "fire." The process is quite rapid, about 50 meters per second in some axons, and resembles the passage of an electric current down a wire.

Axonal Conduction

This "axonal conduction" is frequently described as an "all-or-none" process: an impulse either passes down the axon or it does not. There is no in-between situation. Moreover, the ionic basis of impulse flow down an axon (including the identity of the ions involved) is the same for all neurons in the brain. Thus, a drug that interfered with axonal conduction might interrupt impulse flow of virtually *all* neurons in the brain, with little in the way of subtle discrimination between them. Drugs used as local anesthetics block axonal conduction wherever they are injected, but no known psychoactive drugs act by blocking axonal conduction in the brain. Although agents like novocaine are a blessing to dental patients, such compounds are not generally useful for purposes of modulating brain function.

When an impulse reaches a nerve ending, the "message" is passed along to the adjacent neuron. This event is the key to most information processing in the brain and, not surprisingly, to the actions and effects of psychotropic drugs. For many years scientists thought that the electrical impulse passing down the axon simply jumped the gap from the nerve ending to the adjacent neuronal cells. Only in the late 1920s did experimental evidence accumulate to suggest that chemicals might be involved in this process. The concept of chemical neurotransmission was finally accepted as a universal process around the year 1950.

Chemical Neurotransmission

Synaptic Transmission

Early brain researchers did not envision neurons as discrete cells. Instead, they thought the brain was composed of a vast weblike network of nerve processes.

Synapses and Neurotransmitters

This assumption prevailed until the turn of the century, when the brilliant Spanish neuroanatomist Santiago Ramón y Cajal utilized unique stains to visualize microscopic brain structure more precisely than had been possible in the past. The stains showed that axons did come to discrete endings that separated one nerve cell from the next. Cajal introduced the "neuron doctrine," postulating what we now take for granted: that the brain is composed of a vast number of separate neurons which somehow are able to communicate with each other.

More recent research has clarified the specific mechanisms of neurotransmission and shown it to be a chemical process (see the illustration below). At the nerve ending, the incoming electrical impulse triggers the release of a chemical called a neurotransmitter that diffuses across the gap, or synapse, between the nerve ending and the adjacent neuronal cell. When the neurotransmitter reaches the adjacent cell, it either speeds or slows that cell's rate of firing—shortening or lengthening the intervals between the cell's firing—depending on whether it is an "excitatory" or an "inhibitory" neurotransmitter.

Most neurotransmitters are synthesized within the nerve ending from which they are released. However, some neurotransmitters are partially synthesized in the main body of the cell and then transported down the axon to the nerve ending. Like most specialized chemicals in the body, neurotransmitters are constructed from precursor chemicals that are abundant in the body and employed for diverse purposes. The common dietary amino acids are the precur-

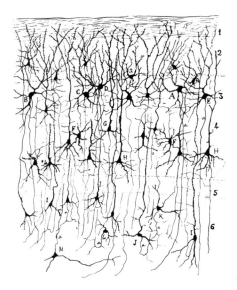

A drawing by Santiago Ramón y Cajal of Golgi-stained nerve tissue as seen under the microscope. Numbers identify cellular layers, and letters differentiate neurons.

Note:

The arrival of the electrical impulse causes the synaptic vesicles in the nerve ending to merge with the cell's outer membrane and spill their load of neurotransmitter into the synaptic cleft. The neurotransmitter molecules diffuse across the synapse and bind to specific receptors in the membrane of the adjacent neuron.

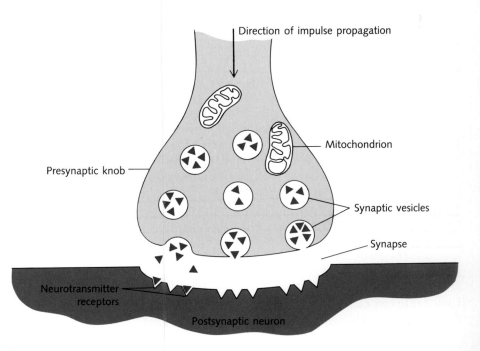

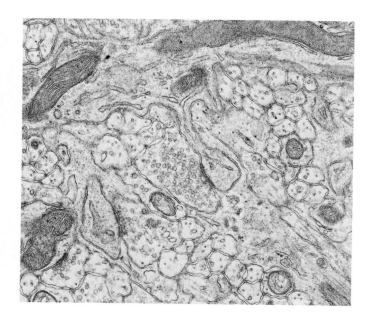

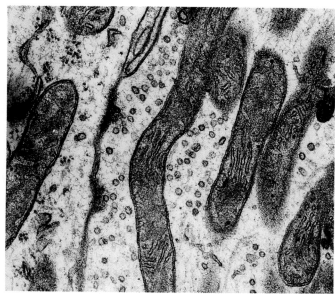

Synaptic vesicles - store neurotransmitters

sors for many neurotransmitters, each of which is built from its precursors through a series of discrete enzymatic steps. (An enzyme is a protein molecule that causes a specific chemical reaction to occur to one or more other molecules. The enzyme itself usually remains unchanged at the reaction's end.) Once synthesized, neurotransmitters are stored in small spherical structures, called synaptic vesicles, within the nerve ending. When an electrical impulse reaches the nerve ending, the synaptic vesicles fuse with the outer membrane of the nerve ending and spill their entire load of neurotransmitters into the synaptic gap.

Once within the synapse, a neurotransmitter molecule faces any number of possible fates. For the purposes of synaptic transmission, the most important outcome is for transmitters to diffuse across the synapse and bind to specific receptor sites on the dendrites of the postsynaptic neuron. The receptors are membrane proteins tailor-made to recognize the neurotransmitter molecules, much as a lock "recognizes" the proper key. The interaction of neurotransmitter with receptor confers specificity on the synaptic process: a neurotransmitter cannot influence a cell that lacks receptors for it; hence, only certain neurons will be affected by certain neurotransmitters. Cells with larger numbers of receptors for a particular transmitter will respond more vigorously than cells with fewer receptors. In ways that are poorly understood, the neurotransmitter-receptor interaction triggers an opening or closing of sodium, potassium, or chloride channels in the synaptic membrane. It is the passage of

Left Tissue from the cerebellar cortex of a rat, at a magnification of 54,000 diameters. A dendritic spine makes contact with a nerve terminal, visible in transverse section (the synaptic vesicles within the axon are also visible). The dark, fuzzy area of contact is the synapse. *Right* Mitochondria are visible within the nerve terminal, where they generate the energy needed for synaptic transmission.

This is the simplest model of receptor binding in which the receptor directly opens, or directly blocks, an ion channel. Other types of receptor mechanisms involve G proteins and cyclic AMP, as illustrated on page 13.

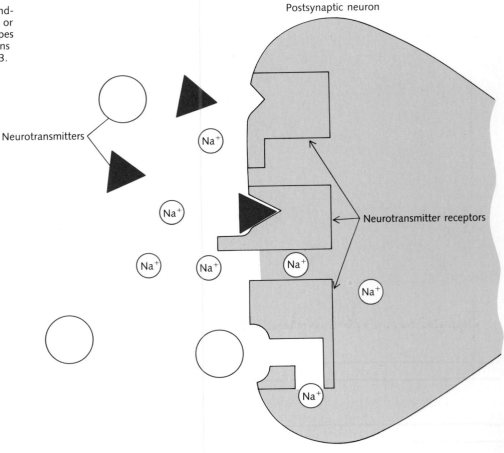

Postsynaptic neuron

Neurotransmitters

Na⁺

Neurotransmitter receptors

sodium and other ions through the membranes, or else a blockade of their movement, that results in either excitation or inhibition of the cell. (Note, however, that these synaptic ion channels are quite distinct from the axonal sodium channels discussed earlier.) Whether excitation or inhibition takes place depends on the chemical nature of the particular neurotransmitter, the type of receptor that recognizes it, and the type of ion channel linked to the receptor. These relationships are summarized in the diagram above and on the facing page.

Synaptic transmission is rapid and brief. As soon as the neurotransmitter interacts with its receptor, it is whisked away, clearing the field for the next burst of transmitter molecules to cross the synapse and initiate a new neuronal impulse. Several inactivation mechanisms have been identified and are illustrated on page 12. Some kinds of neurotransmitters are destroyed by enzymes

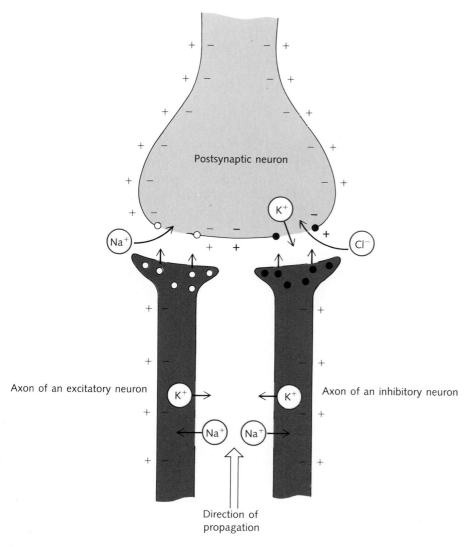

Comparison of excitatory and inhibitory neurotransmission. When the excitatory neurotransmitter binds to postsynaptic receptors, a local depolarization of the post-synaptic membrane is produced through an increased permeability to positive ions, especially Na^+. In contrast, the inhibitory transmitter causes a local hyperpolarization by enhancing the passage of smaller ions like K^+ and Cl^-.

located in the vicinity of the synapse. More frequently, however, neurotransmitters are pumped back into the axon that released them. The nerve-ending membrane has a site that recognizes its particular type of neurotransmitter and activates an energy-requiring enzymatic system that sucks the transmitter back into the axon's interior. This reuptake mechanism also provides a way for the nerve ending to conserve neurotransmitter molecules and use them again and again. In some situations, glia make use of a similar pump to remove transmitter molecules from the synaptic space.

After a neurotransmitter is recognized by a receptor site on the postsynaptic neuron, a number of other events take place. Certain cellular alterations—

Neurotransmitter molecules are disposed of in various ways. Some are degraded by enzymes (1); others are pumped back into the neuron that released them (2) or are pumped into glia (3). Some kinds of neurotransmitters simply diffuse away from the synapse (4).

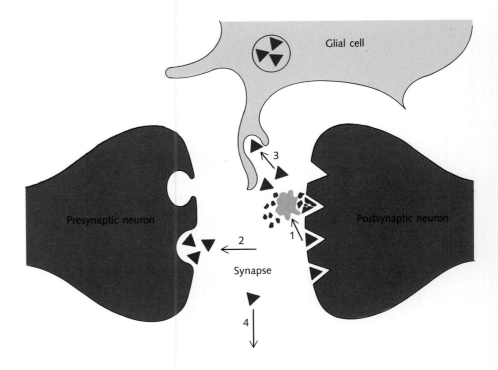

usually referred to as "second messengers," because they intervene between the original message and its ultimate effect on the nerve cell—must "translate" the receptor's recognition of the neurotransmitter into an alteration in the firing rate and general metabolic activity of the neuron. Some neurotransmitter receptors are linked directly to particular ion channels that act as second messengers. In many instances, however, biochemical systems intervene to carry the message. The best-known chemical second messenger is called cyclic AMP (adenosine -3'5'-*mono*phosphate); its role in neurotransmission is illustrated on the facing page. Many neurotransmitters stimulate the formation of cyclic AMP from its precursor, ATP (adenosine *tri*phosphate), which is also the major source of energy in the body. In these systems, recognition of a neurotransmitter by its receptor indirectly stimulates the activity of adenylate cyclase, the enzyme that makes cyclic AMP from ATP.

The effect of the transmitter-receptor interaction on adenylate cyclase activity is mediated by yet another link in the chain of communications: certain proteins, referred to as GTP-binding proteins because they bind the nucleotide GTP (guanosine *tri*phosphate), help translate the receptor's recognition of the neurotransmitter into a change in the neuron's level of adenylate cyclase activity. While some neurotransmitters enhance adenylate cyclase, others influence cellular activity by *depressing* the activity of adenylate cyclase. Whether a

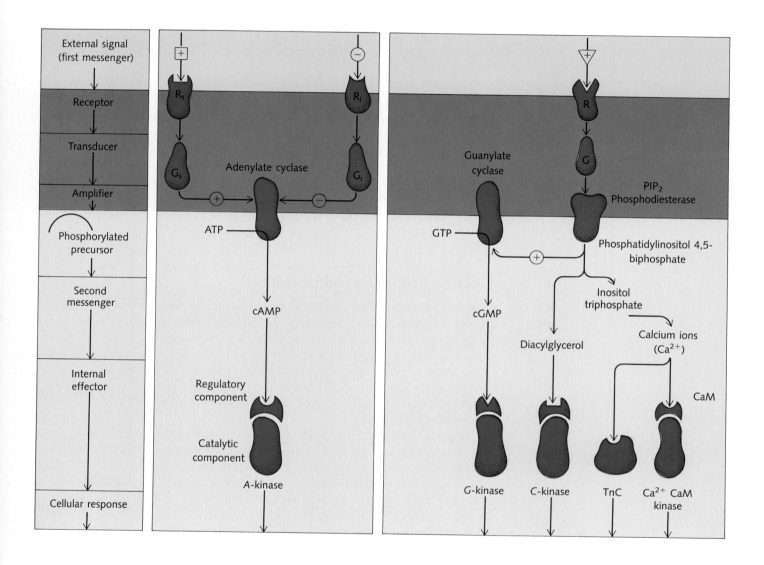

External signal (first messenger)	
Receptor	
Transducer	
Amplifier	
Phosphorylated precursor	
Second messenger	
Internal effector	
Cellular response	

Adenylate cyclase

R_s R_i G_s G_i

ATP

cAMP

Regulatory component

Catalytic component

A-kinase

Guanylate cyclase

R G

PIP$_2$ Phosphodiesterase

GTP

Phosphatidylinositol 4,5-biphosphate

cGMP

Inositol triphosphate

Diacylglycerol

Calcium ions (Ca^{2+})

CaM

G-kinase C-kinase TnC Ca^{2+} CaM kinase

given neurotransmitter stimulates or inhibits adenylate cyclase depends on the type of GTP-binding protein linked to the receptor. Two distinct GTP-binding proteins have been seen to regulate cyclic AMP formation: one is specific for stimulation of adenylate cyclase, and the other is specific for its inhibition.

Cyclic AMP stimulates the phosphorylation of certain proteins in cells; this means that phosphate ions become attached to the proteins, a process thought to be the key link in the cyclic AMP second-messenger system. Different proteins are phosphorylated in different target cells. The phosphorylated proteins act directly upon the nerve cell's ion channels. The ultimate purpose of the

First- and second-messenger events. The sequence of events is summarized at the left, highlighting the similarities between two of the known pathways.

second-messenger system is to phosphorylate a particular protein and thereby regulate a particular cellular function. In this way, the "message" of the neurotransmitter is expressed.

Another equally important second-messenger system is the more recently characterized phosphoinositide cycle. Phosphoinositides are chemicals that have both sugars and lipids in their structure. They are synthesized in a complex series of enzymatic reactions, some of which cause certain proteins inside the cells to be phosphorylated. In this way, the phosphoinositide cycle and the cyclic AMP system perform a similar second-messenger function, the phosphorylation of particular proteins. Both the cyclic AMP system and the phosphoinositide system are highly complex, and neither is well understood by researchers. The present state of knowledge is depicted in the figure on the previous page.

How Drugs Affect Neurotransmitters

Drugs can influence the process of synaptic transmission in a number of ways; some are illustrated on the facing page. For example, because all neurotransmitters must be synthesized from precursor molecules in the presence of particular enzymes, a drug that inhibited one of those enzymes would impede the formation of neurotransmitters. Clinical medicine makes use of numerous drugs that act in this way. For instance, certain drugs that treat high blood pressure block the formation of norepinephrine, a neurotransmitter that elevates blood pressure.

Some drugs interfere with the storage of neurotransmitters by causing them to leak out of synaptic vesicles. Once out of the vesicles, the transmitters are degraded by enzymes, leaving the nerve ending devoid of messenger molecules. Reserpine, a tranquilizer that also lowers blood pressure, is such a drug; it acts by interfering with the storage of norepinephrine.

Other drugs affect the release of neurotransmitters from nerve endings. Some of these compounds resemble the neurotransmitter in chemical structure and are thus able to slip into the vesicles in place of the transmitter molecules, virtually pushing the transmitters out into the synaptic cleft. Amphetamines act in this way to release norepinephrine and a related transmitter called dopamine in the brain. In contrast, drugs like bretylium, an antihypertensive agent, block the release process itself.

Some therapeutic agents act by inhibiting enzymes that degrade neurotransmitter molecules, thus augmenting levels of the transmitter and facilitating synaptic transmission. Certain antidepressants inhibit the enzyme monoamine oxidase, which degrades transmitters responsible for mood regulation. Other drugs facilitate synaptic transmission by blocking the reuptake inactivation process. Examples include the most widely used antidepressants, known as tricyclic antidepressants.

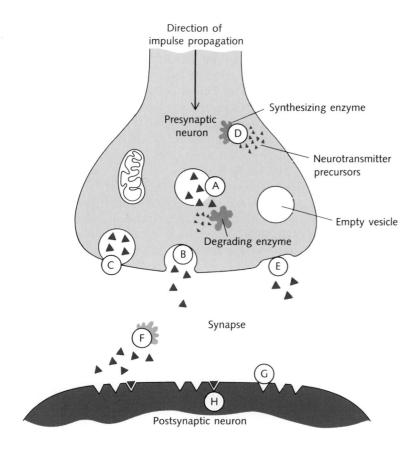

Direction of
impulse propagation

Presynaptic
neuron

Synthesizing enzyme

Neurotransmitter
precursors

Empty vesicle

Degrading enzyme

Synapse

Postsynaptic neuron

Drugs affect neurotransmission by causing neurotransmitter molecules to leak out of synaptic vesicles (A); crowding neurotransmitters out of storage vesicles (B); blocking release of neurotransmitter into the synapse (C); inhibiting enzymes that synthesize neurotransmitters (D); blocking neurotransmitter reuptake (E); blocking enzymes that degrade neurotransmitters (F); or binding to the receptor and either mimicking or blocking neurotransmitters (G). Hypothetical drug H interferes with or facilitates second-messenger activity.

Finally, perhaps the most common therapeutically relevant activity of a psychoactive drug is to influence the neurotransmitter receptor. Some drugs bear a chemical resemblance to the neurotransmitter and mimic its effects at receptors. Others may occupy the receptor without causing any second-messenger response within the nerve. Such drugs do not alter neuronal firing directly; rather they block the effects of neurotransmitter molecules by blocking their access to receptors.

When scientists investigate the way in which a drug influences a particular neurotransmitter, they are also interested in knowing *where* in the brain that particular drug action takes place. Different parts of the brain have different functions, and neurons are organized into circuits that direct messages to the different regions in an ordered and meaningful way. The cerebral cortex, for example, is the seat of perception and logical thinking, as well as of certain aspects of motor activity; the extrapyramidal areas, beneath the cortex, integrate information to bring about movement, which the cerebellum coordi-

Chapter 1

nates; the limbic system lends emotional coloring to our perceptions and thoughts, alerting us to those that deserve most attention. Some of the important regions within the brain are depicted in the drawing opposite.

All the different modes of drug action in the brain have been identified in connection with a few transmitters that have been extensively characterized, and it is only recently that scientists have come to realize there are at least fifty distinct neurotransmitters carrying messages in the brain. Who knows how many more kinds of drug-neurotransmitter interactions have yet to be detected and analyzed? Until the mid-1970s no more than five neurotransmitters had been studied in detail. Virtually all the drugs used in psychiatry today act through one of this handful of transmitter molecules. The forty-five or more transmitters discovered in recent years are equally useful targets for the design of new psychoactive agents. Drug companies just have not had time to conduct all the basic and clinical research required to develop a therapeutically valuable substance. Considering the immense impact that the present generation of drugs has had upon the treatment of emotional and neurological disease, the extent of control scientists are likely to achieve over disease processes in the next few decades is truly awe-inspiring.

Acetylcholine as a Model Neurotransmitter

The general features of neurotransmission outlined above are exemplified by the activity of acetylcholine, a well-characterized substance that was the first neurotransmitter to be identified; in fact, investigations involving this substance provided the first solid evidence that chemical neurotransmission exists. Acetylcholine also demonstrates the important interplay between drugs and neurotransmitters in developing therapeutic agents, elucidating brain function, and explaining the symptoms of a major brain disorder.

The role of acetylcholine as a neurotransmitter was initially discovered not in the brain but in the heart. In 1921, Otto Loewi, a German pharmacologist and physiologist, was experimenting with the vagus nerve, the major nerve regulating heart function. The vagus has its cell bodies in the lower brainstem and sends axons down into various organs of the body, including the salivary glands, the intestines, the lungs, and the heart. Loewi, interested in how the vagus slowed contractions of heart muscle, asked, do electrical impulses passing down the vagus nerve simply continue directly into the heart muscle, or does the vagus release some chemical that is the active agent regulating the heart? His experimental approach, illustrated on page 20, was quite straightforward. He placed a frog's heart, with the vagus nerve attached, in a bathing solution similar to the extracellular fluids of the body, and then he electrically stimulated the nerve. He knew that vigorous stimulation of the vagus slows and even stops the beating of the heart. When he had stimulated the nerve enough to stop the frog's heart from beating, Loewi took the fluid that bathed the stimulated heart and applied it to a second frog's heart. The second heart

Facing page Important anatomical divisions of the brain. These include the cerebral cortex, which carries out the "highest" brain functions, such as reflection and reasoning; the thalamus, a "funnel" that transmits sensory information to the cerebral cortex; the cerebellum, which governs voluntary motor control; and the midbrain, pons, and medulla oblongata, which govern basic life functions, such as breathing and heartbeat.

16

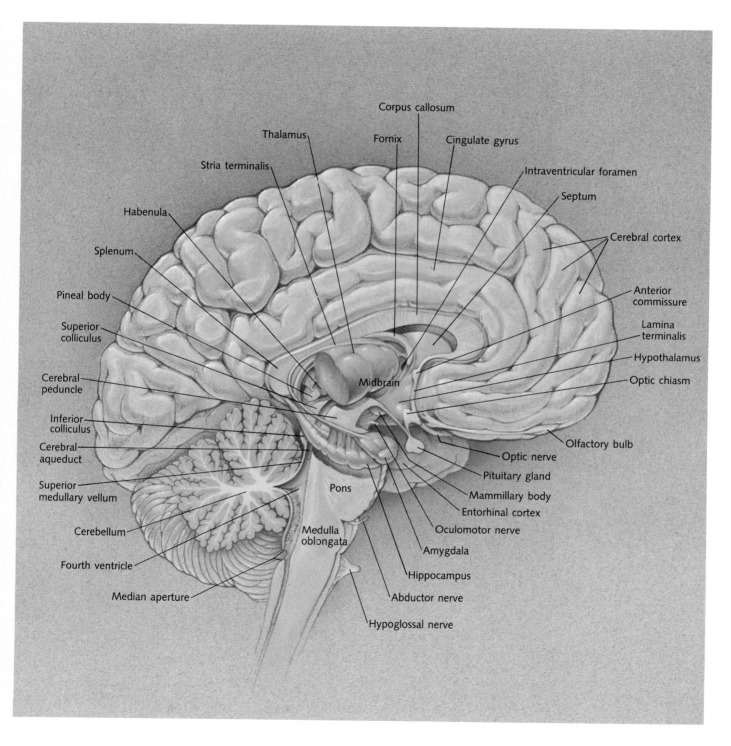

Some prominent neurotransmitters in the brain

Acetylcholine | The first known neurotransmitter, discovered in the 1920s. It is the neurotransmitter at nerve-muscle connections for all the voluntary muscles of the body as well as at many of the involuntary (autonomic) nervous system synapses. Despite its long history, the exact role of acetylcholine neurons in the brain is unclear.

Norepinephrine | One of the two major catecholamine neurotransmitters and the second known transmitter, having been characterized in the 1930s. It was discovered as the transmitter of the sympathetic nerves of the autonomic nervous system which mediate emergency responses, such as acceleration of the heart, dilatation of the bronchi, and elevation of blood pressure.

Dopamine | Another catecholamine neurotransmitter, discovered in 1958 as a major transmitter in the corpus striatum, a part of the brain regulating motor behavior. Destruction of the dopamine neurons in the corpus striatum is responsible for the symptoms of Parkinson's disease, such as rigidity and tremor. Blockade of the actions of dopamine in other brain regions accounts for the therapeutic activities of antischizophrenic drugs.

Serotonin | The transmitter of a discrete group of neurons that all have cell bodies located in the raphe nuclei of the brain stem. Changes in the activity of serotonin neurons are related to the actions of psychedelic drugs.

Enkephalins | Composed of two peptides, each containing five amino acids. The enkephalins are neurotransmitters that were discovered as the normally occurring substances which act upon opiate receptors. Thus, enkephalins can mimic the effects of opiates. Enkephalin neurons are localized to areas of the brain which regulate functions that are influenced by opiate drugs.

Substance P | A peptide containing eleven amino acids. It is a major transmitter of sensory neurons which convey pain sensation from the periphery, especially the skin, into the spinal cord. Opiates relieve pain in part by blocking the release of substance P. Substance P is also found in numerous brain regions.

GABA (gamma-aminobutyric acid) | This is one of the amino acid transmitters in the brain. It has no known function besides serving as a neurotransmitter and occurs almost exclusively in the brain. GABA reduces the firing of neurons and so is an inhibitory neurotransmitter. It is the transmitter at 25 to 40 percent of all synapses in the brain, and so, quantitatively, it may be the predominant transmitter of the brain.

Glycine	Besides its roles as a conventional amino acid in protein synthesis and general metabolism, glycine serves as an inhibitory neurotransmitter in small neurons in the spinal cord and brain stem. Here it is a transmitter at 30 to 40 percent of synapses and quantitatively is more prominent than GABA, which in turn predominates in higher centers such as the cerebral cortex.
Glutamic acid	One of the major amino acids in general metabolism and protein synthesis, glutamic acid is also a neurotransmitter. It stimulates neurons to fire and is probably the principal excitatory neurotransmitter in the brain. Glutamic acid appears to be the neurotransmitter of the major neuronal pathway that connects the cerebral cortex and the corpus striatum. It is also the transmitter of the granule cells, which are the most numerous neurons in the cerebellum. There is some evidence that glutamic acid is the principal neurotransmitter of the visual pathway. No drugs are yet known to exert their effects via interactions with glutamic acid.
Histamine	In addition to its roles in the periphery in allergic conditions and in regulating acid secretion by the stomach, histamine is a neurotransmitter in the brain. It is most highly concentrated in areas of the brain that regulate emotional behavior, and its localization is roughly similar to that of norepinephrine. It is unclear whether the central effects of antihistamine drugs, such as somnolence, relate to actions at brain histamine receptors.

promptly ceased beating. Loewi reasoned that when the vagus nerve was stimulated, some chemical must have been released that could reproduce the ability of nerve impulses to slow and stop the beating of the heart. Within five years of his initial experiment, Loewi was able to prove that acetylcholine is the substance released by the vagus nerve to inhibit the beating of the heart.

Acetylcholine is synthesized in nerves by a single enzymatic step that was not characterized until ten years after Loewi's work. This enzymatic step links together two ubiquitous body chemicals: choline (especially important in fat metabolism, and an ingredient of many foodstuffs) and acetyl coenzyme A, an activated form of acetic acid (the chief acid of vinegar and a central component in the chain of reactions that turns food into energy). The enzyme is called choline acetyltransferase, and it occurs in a freely mobile form in the cytoplasm of acetylcholine-containing nerve endings. Once synthesized, acetylcholine is

Loewi's discovery of the first-known neuro-transmitter. The "donor" heart (D), with vagus nerve attached, was bathed in saline solution, which was then routed to the isolated "recipient" heart (R). Stimulation (S) of the vagus caused the donor heart to slow; 15 seconds later, the recipient heart slowed, too, in reaction to the acetylcholine that the donor heart had released into the bathing solution. Time (T) is shown in 5-second intervals.

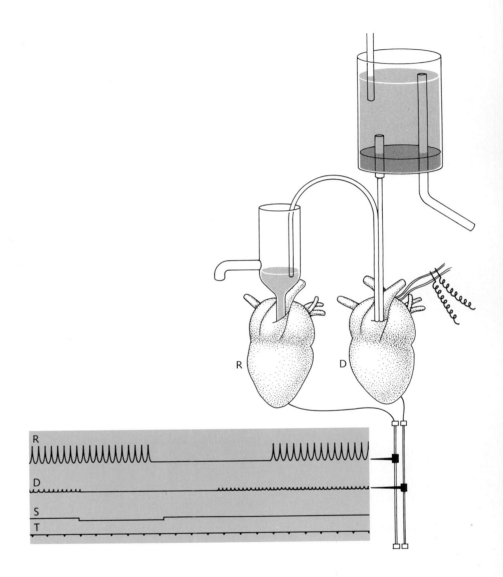

stored in synaptic vesicles until an impulse traveling down the axon triggers its release.

After acetylcholine has crossed the synapse and interacted with a receptor, its effects are terminated by another enzyme, acetylcholinesterase. As the drawing on page 22 illustrates, this enzyme is located adjacent to the receptors, where it can act immediately to break the bond between choline and acetic acid. The choline released in this fashion is pumped back into the nerve ending that originally released the acetylcholine and is thus conserved for reinsertion

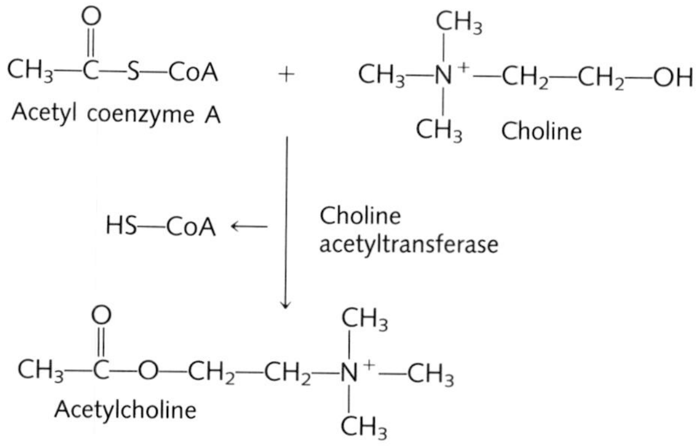

$$CH_3-\overset{\overset{\displaystyle O}{\|}}{C}-S-CoA \quad + \quad CH_3-\overset{\overset{\displaystyle CH_3}{|}}{\underset{\underset{\displaystyle CH_3}{|}}{N^+}}-CH_2-CH_2-OH$$

Acetyl coenzyme A   Choline

$$HS-CoA \leftarrow \quad \begin{array}{l}\text{Choline}\\\text{acetyltransferase}\end{array}$$

$$CH_3-\overset{\overset{\displaystyle O}{\|}}{C}-O-CH_2-CH_2-\overset{\overset{\displaystyle CH_3}{|}}{\underset{\underset{\displaystyle CH_3}{|}}{N^+}}-CH_3$$

Acetylcholine

Biosynthesis of acetylcholine from choline and acetyl coenzyme A.

into new acetylcholine molecules. (Interestingly, this enzymatic mechanism for inactivating acetylcholine is something of an exception to the general rule. Most neurotransmitters in the brain are inactivated by neuronal reuptake, but scientists have been unable to find a similar acetylcholine uptake system in nerve endings.)

Acetylcholine serves as a neurotransmitter for 10 to 15 percent of neurons in the human nervous system. It is the transmitter for all the nerves that act on voluntary muscles like those of the arms and legs, and it is also a transmitter for nerves to most glands in the body.

The importance of acetylcholine as a neurotransmitter and of acetylcholinesterase as its inactivator is evident from the effects of chemicals that interact with them. For instance, acetylcholine is present in insects as well as in humans and all other members of the animal kingdom, and for many years inhibitors of acetylcholinesterase have been the most widely used insecticides in the world. By inhibiting acetylcholinesterase, these insecticides cause acetylcholine to accumulate in the insect's nervous system, causing toxicity via mechanisms that are not yet clear. The crucial role of acetylcholinesterase in human nervous

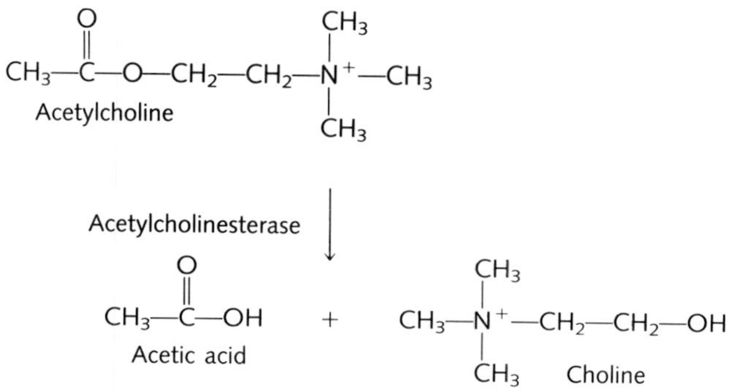

$$CH_3-\overset{\overset{\displaystyle O}{\|}}{C}-O-CH_2-CH_2-\overset{\overset{\displaystyle CH_3}{|}}{\underset{\underset{\displaystyle CH_3}{|}}{N^+}}-CH_3$$

Acetylcholine

$$\text{Acetylcholinesterase} \downarrow$$

$$CH_3-\overset{\overset{\displaystyle O}{\|}}{C}-OH \quad + \quad CH_3-\overset{\overset{\displaystyle CH_3}{|}}{\underset{\underset{\displaystyle CH_3}{|}}{N^+}}-CH_2-CH_2-OH$$

Acetic acid   Choline

Degradation of acetylcholine by acetylcholinesterase.

Acetylcholine (ACh) activity at a synapse.

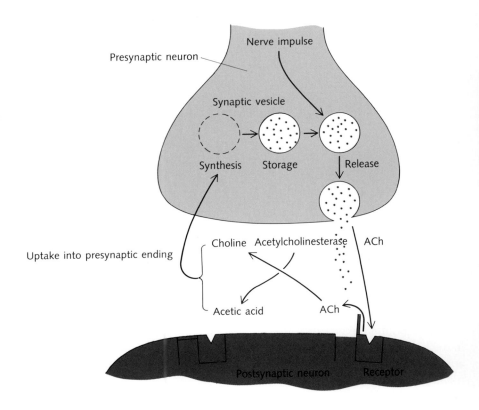

Facing page Acetylcholine pathways. Those projecting to the hippocampus and cerebral cortex play a major role in memory functions.

function is evident from the toxicity of these insecticides to small children, who all too frequently ingest them by accident. Because acetylcholine is the transmitter of nerve impulses to the diaphragm, acetylcholinesterase-inhibiting insecticides can paralyze a young child's breathing apparatus.

In addition to its functions as a neurotransmitter to the heart and other peripheral organs, acetylcholine is also a neurotransmitter in the brain itself. In fact, it is one of the principal neurotransmitters in the cerebral cortex. Some of the acetylcholine-containing nerves there are quite short, with cell bodies, axons, and nerve endings all confined within the cortex. These nerves are thought to handle the complex information processing necessary for "higher" mental functions, such as reflective thinking. Other acetylcholine-containing nerves are much longer, with cell bodies located outside the cerebral cortex in an area called the basal nucleus of Meynert and axons extending throughout the cortex. The basal nucleus was an enigmatic structure until research in the late 1970s showed that it contained acetylcholine neurons. The combination of that discovery and recent findings in pharmacology and medicine has enabled scientists to predict some remarkable connections between acetylcholine, brain anatomy, and human behavior.

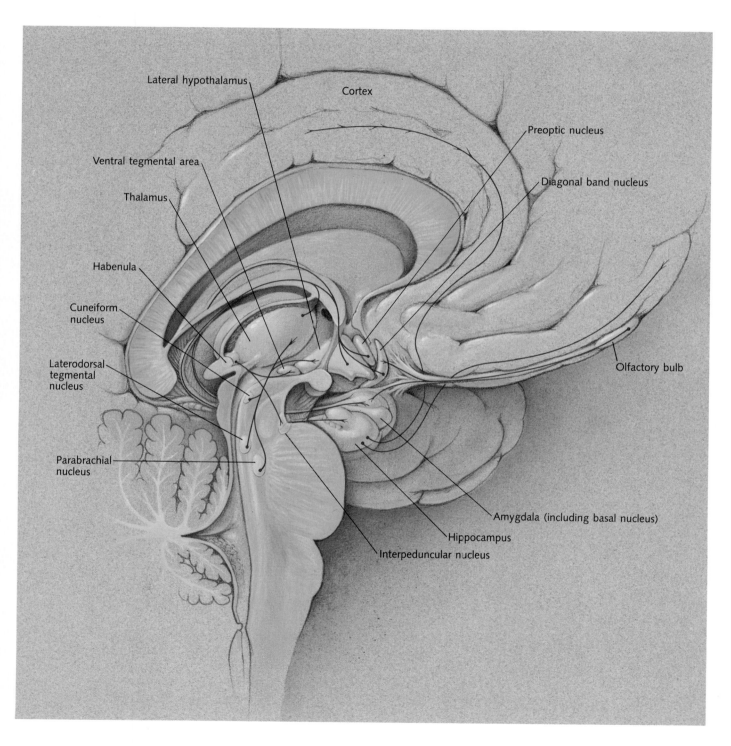

Lateral hypothalamus

Cortex

Preoptic nucleus

Diagonal band nucleus

Ventral tegmental area

Thalamus

Habenula

Cuneiform nucleus

Laterodorsal tegmental nucleus

Olfactory bulb

Parabrachial nucleus

Amygdala (including basal nucleus)

Hippocampus

Interpeduncular nucleus

The medicinal properties of certain drugs that block acetylcholine receptors were recognized and employed in medical practice for hundreds of years before anyone had ever heard of neurotransmitters. Extracts of the belladonna plant, for example, have been used since the days of Hippocrates to treat intestinal disturbances, slowing down intestinal contractions and reducing acid secretion in the stomach. In the Middle Ages, these belladonna alkaloids were also used as poisons; lethal doses were observed to cause memory loss, disorientation, and destruction of other mental faculties before the victim finally succumbed. In fact, Carolus Linnaeus, the founder of modern botanical nomenclature, named the plant *Atropa belladonna* after Atropos, the oldest of the Three Fates, who was said to cut the thread of life after her sisters had spun and measured it.

In the mid-1800s, atropine, the active ingredient of the belladonna plant, was isolated and shown to block the ability of vagus nerve stimulation to slow the heart. In the 1930s, it was proved that this action is due to the ability of atropine to block a receptor for acetylcholine. The atropine-acetylcholine connection suggested that, if one of the most striking symptoms of atropine overdose is loss of memory, then acetylcholine nerves in the brain might have something to do with memory processes. A heartbreaking neurological disorder known as Alzheimer's disease provides an "experiment of nature" to help test this hypothesis.

Acetylcholine and Alzheimer's Disease

Alzheimer's disease is a disorder that primarily affects the elderly and is associated with memory loss. Sometimes the memory loss experienced by elderly people is caused by blood clots or hemorrhages in cerebral vessels; more commonly, however, Alzheimer's disease is the cause of senile dementia, the mental deterioration that frequently accompanies old age.

In searching for possible biochemical abnormalities in the brains of patients with senile dementia, researchers measured levels of numerous neurotransmitters. When postmortem brains of patients with Alzheimer's disease and of age-matched individuals with normal mental function were analyzed, the levels of most neurotransmitters were found to be quite normal. Only acetylcholine and the enzyme that catalyzes its formation were found to be greatly reduced in the brains of patients with Alzheimer's disease. Considering that ingestion of atropine causes memory loss and has been shown to block the neurotransmission of acetylcholine, these postmortem brain studies suggested that an acetylcholine deficiency is responsible for the symptoms of Alzheimer's disease.

If an acetylcholine deficiency were indeed the cause of memory loss in Alzheimer's disease, certain of the acetylcholine neurons might be expected to degenerate in Alzheimer's patients. Researchers next examined the parts of the brain that they knew to be rich in acetylcholine neurons. One of these was the neuronal pathway projecting from the basal nucleus up into the cerebral cor-

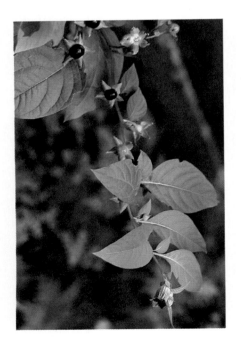

Atropa belladonna, source of the acetylcholine antagonist atropine.

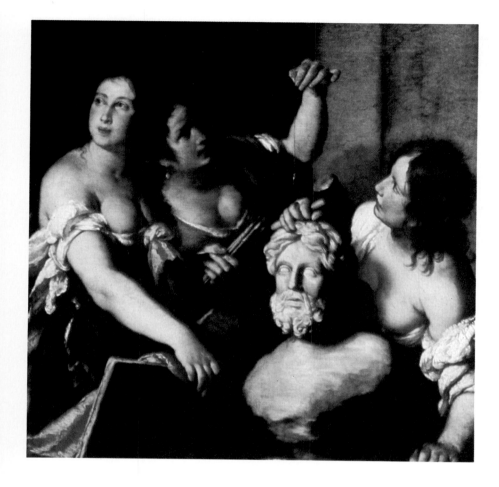

The Three Fates by Bernardo Strozzi. At death, Atropos cuts the thread of life.

tex. Brain specimens of patients who had died with Alzheimer's disease did in fact reveal a massive degeneration of the basal nucleus. Most other neuronal groups looked relatively normal. This suggests that neurons of the basal nucleus regulate mental processes such as memory that are impaired in Alzheimer's disease.

Researchers are now faced with the challenge of developing drugs that might alleviate Alzheimer's symptoms. Some scientists have tried to replace the missing acetylcholine by treating patients with large doses of the precursor choline. This approach has been relatively ineffective because, as was mentioned above, patients with Alzheimer's disease are also deficient in choline acetyltransferase, the enzyme that synthesizes acetylcholine. Choline acetyltransferase is normally stored in the acetylcholine nerves that degenerate in Alzheimer's disease.

Chemical structure of atropine.

Chapter 1

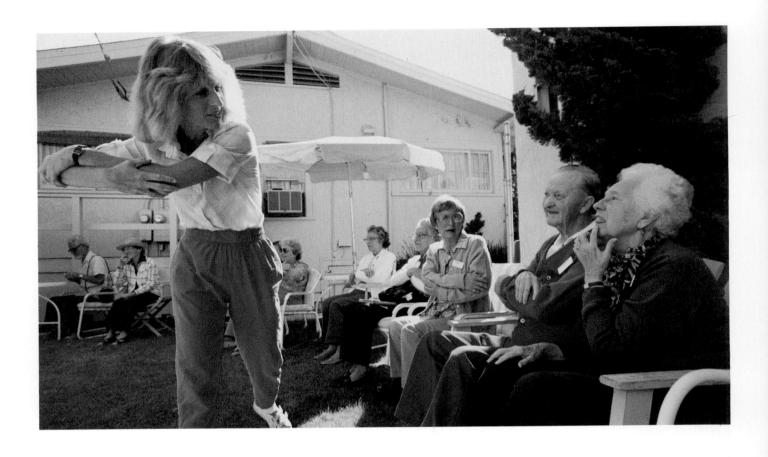

An exercise class for Alzheimer victims.

An alternative approach might be to develop drugs that mimic acetylcholine at its receptors. Acetylcholine itself cannot be used for at least two reasons: (1) it is rapidly destroyed in the body by enzymes, primarily acetylcholinesterase, the enzyme that normally inactivates it at synapses; and (2) even if it were not destroyed, acetylcholine administered by mouth or injection is unlikely to reach its target organ, the brain. To protect the brain from noxious chemicals that circulate in the blood, nature has evolved a "blood-brain barrier" that keeps electrically charged molecules from passing out of the blood and into the brain (see the diagram on page 27). Acetylcholine is a highly charged molecule that would have great difficulty passing through this barrier after being ingested or injected. Accordingly, chemists in the pharmaceutical industry are currently attempting to synthesize derivatives of acetylcholine that are metabolically stable and less electrically charged so they may be capable of crossing into the brain. So far, no therapeutic agents based on this model have yet been evaluated in humans, but research in this area has only recently commenced. Many scientists are hopeful that before the end of the twentieth century effec-

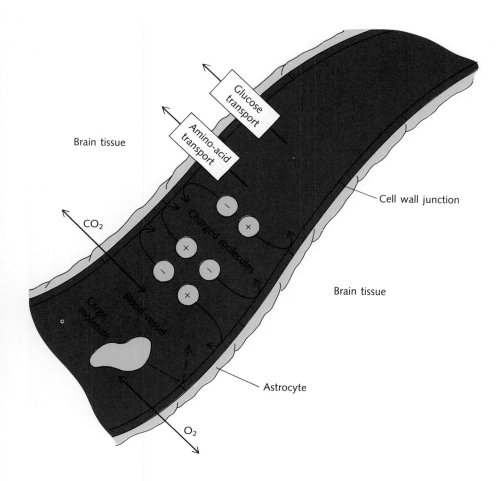

Brain tissue

Glucose transport

Amino-acid transport

CO_2

Charged molecules

Blood vessel

Large molecule

O_2

Cell wall junction

Brain tissue

Astrocyte

The blood-brain barrier. Tight cell-wall junctions and a coating of astrocytes around the blood vessel prevent large or charged molecules from passing out of the bloodstream and into the brain. Special carrier mechanisms transport nutrient molecules, while small neutral molecules pass freely, depending on their relative concentrations on opposite sides of the membrane.

tive therapy will be available for the millions of victims suffering from Alzheimer's dementia.

This is only one example of how pharmacologists and neurologists have collaborated to uncover an important aspect of brain function and to expedite the development of new therapeutic drugs. In the following six chapters, we will examine six groups of powerful psychoactive drugs: opiates, antischizophrenics, antidepressants, stimulants, tranquilizers, and psychedelic drugs. We will study the effects these powerful compounds exert on synaptic transmission in the brain, and we will see how identifying their mechanisms and sites of action leads to major advances both in the safety and effectiveness of drug therapy and in our understanding of how the human brain perceives the world, plans for the future, sleeps, wakes, fears, desires—and, sometimes, goes insane.

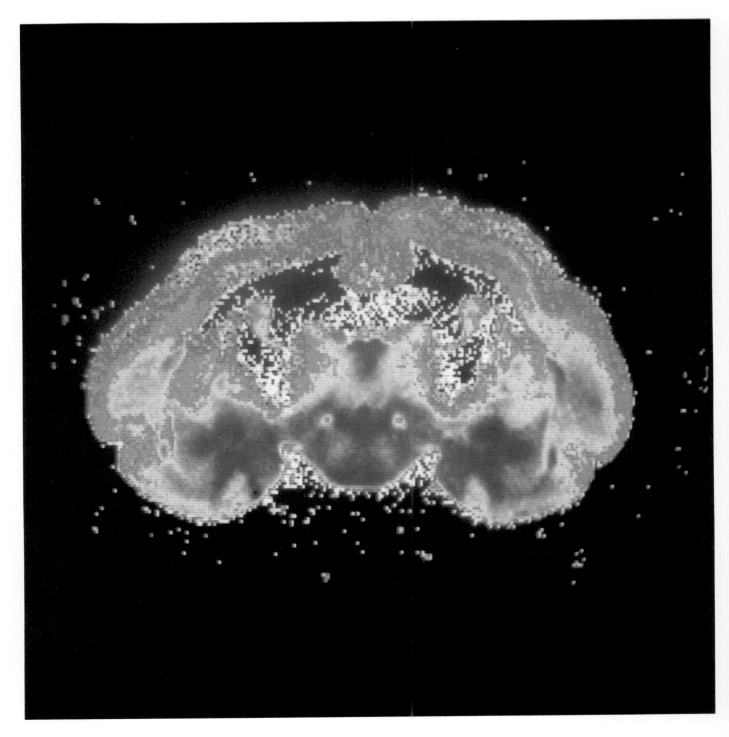

28

2 | Opiates

Thomas Sydenham, perhaps the greatest physician of the late seventeenth century, once commented, "I cannot forebear mentioning with gratitude the goodness of the Supreme Being, who has supplied afflicted mankind with opiates for their relief; no other remedy being equally powerful to overcome a great number of diseases, or to eradicate them effectually." Historically, opiates have been among the most important agents in medicine. The second-century Greek physician Galen, revered for centuries as the highest authority in medicine, administered opium to relieve the pain of headaches, gallbladder maladies, colic, and kidney stones. Galen also employed opium as a calming agent to ease the agitated breathing of patients suffering from asthma and congestive heart failure. Despite exhaustive efforts over the past hundred years, no one has succeeded in finding other pain-relieving agents nearly so powerful.

At the same time, opiates are the classic examples of the addictive substance, exacting a massive toll on society. Their devastating effects are not easily quantified, but some statistics have been gathered, and these paint a bleak picture. For example, each year in the United States, several billion dollars of property are lost in burglaries to support heroin habits. If we could understand how opiates cause addiction, we might thereby attain insight into the addictive processes of all sorts of dependence-producing drugs and find ways to develop agents that prevent dependence from occurring. Similarly, if we understood how opiates act in the brain to relieve pain and induce warm feelings of tranquility and well-being, we might be able to design substances that could reproduce these beneficial effects without creating the tolerance and dependence so devastating to drug addicts and their communities.

Opiate Use in Western Culture

Opium is an extract of the poppy plant and has probably been used for its psychoactive effects longer than any other agent, except perhaps alcohol. Writ-

Facing page Distribution of opiate receptors in guinea pig brain. Red = highest density of receptors; yellow = moderate density; blue = low density; purple and white = very low densities.

Opium poppies grown for pharmaceutical use.

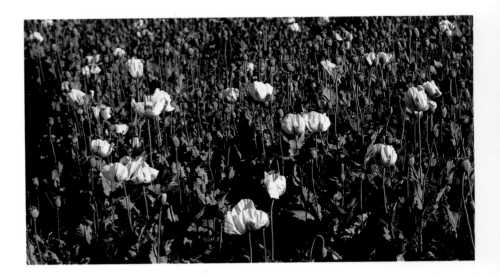

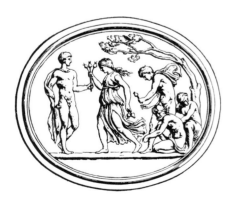

Nix, the Greek goddess of night, dispensing opium poppies. This engraving is based on an antique cameo.

ings that seem to refer to poppy extracts with opiate actions have been found in the area of Sumeria in the Middle East and judged to date from 4000 B.C. The ancient Greeks used opium for its recreational as well as its medicinal effects. In *The Odyssey,* composed in the ninth or eighth century B.C., Homer tells how a plant-derived drug called nepenthe was employed to elicit a feeling of quiet warmth and well-being followed by somnolence and sleep. This description succinctly conveys the nature of the euphoria elicited by opiates, a calm state in contrast to the hyperalert, excited euphoria associated with stimulants such as cocaine or amphetamines. The importance of opium in Roman culture is evident from the fact that Somnus, the Roman god of sleep, is often depicted carrying a container filled with the juice of the poppy plant.

While opium has always been important in medicine, its recreational use in Europe stems from the experiments and writings of the British Romantic authors of the nineteenth century, whose works emphasized the emotional, mystical, imaginative side of human nature. Much of the interest in opium was sparked by Thomas De Quincey, who published an essay, "Confessions of an English Opium-Eater," in 1821. He had first used opium to relieve the pain of a toothache and wrote, "That my pains had vanished was now a trifle in my eyes. . . . Here was the secret of happiness, that which philosophers had disputed for so many ages, at once discovered; happiness might now be bought for a penny, and carried in the waist coat pocket; portable ecstasies might be had corked up in a pint bottle; and peace of mind could be sent down by the mail."

De Quincey started a trend among writers in England, despite the fact that the dangers of opium addiction were by then well known. He convinced the

Take Opium, 1 Ounce

For centuries, opium appeared as a standard ingredient in all sorts of medicinal preparations. Though the drug is known to have been in use long before the common era, the earliest example presented here, the recipe for philonium, was devised in the first century A.D.

Philonium, an ancient Roman prescription for colic or dysentery.
White pepper, ginger, caraway seeds, strained opium and syrup of poppies, the proportion of opium being 1 grain in 36 grains of the confection.

Theriaca, prescribed by Galen for numerous diverse complaints, including poisoning, headaches, deafness, epilepsy, dimness of vision, jaundice, fevers, and leprosy.
Root of Florentine iris, licorice, 12 ounces each; of Arabian costus, Pontic rhubarb, cinquefoil, 6 ounces each; of Ligusticum meum, rhubarb, gentian, 4 ounces each; of birthwort, 2 ounces; herb of scordium, 12 ounces; of lemon grass, horehound, dittany of Crete, calamint, 6 ounces each; . . . of anise, fennel, cress, seseli, thlaspi, amomum, sandwort, 4 ounces each; of carrot, 2 ounces; opium, 24 ounces; . . . of vipers, of sweet flag, 24 ounces each.
Triturate the balsams, resins and gums in a sufficient quantity of wine to form a thin paste, and incorporate the whole with 960 ounces of honey.

Diascordium, formulated in the sixteenth century as a means of preventing the plague.
Cinnamon, cassia wood, scordium, dittany, galbanum, storax, gum arabic, opium, sorrel, gentian, Armenian bole, Lemnian earth, pepper, ginger, and honey.

Dover's powder, a seventeenth-century remedy for gout.
Take opium, 1 ounce; saltpeter and tartar vitriolated, each 4 ounces; liquorice, 1 ounce; ipecacuanha, 1 ounce: Put the saltpeter and tartar into a red hot mortar, stirring till they have done flaming. Then powder very fine. After that, slice in your opium; grind to a powder and mix. Dose, from 40 to 60 or 70 grains in a glass of white wine posset, going to bed, covering up warm, and drinking a quart or three pints of the posset while sweating. In two or three hours at furthest the patient will be free from pain.

poets Samuel Taylor Coleridge and Elizabeth Barrett Browning to try the drug, both of whom subsequently became addicts. (Coleridge's well-known poem *Kubla Khan* describes a vision he experienced while under the influence of opium.) Even in the sixteenth and seventeenth centuries physicians warned of the drug's hazards. For instance, a Dr. John Jones commented, "The effects

Depiction of a Parisian opium den, near the turn of the century.

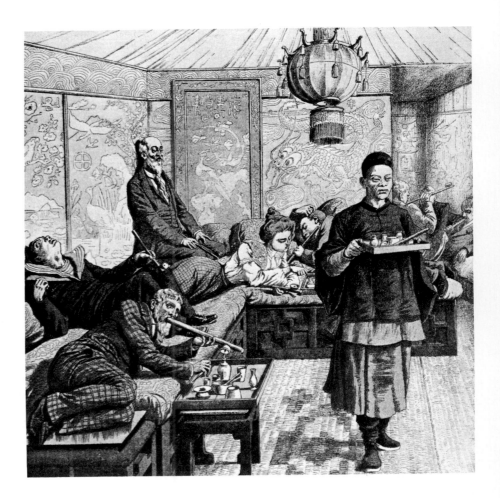

of suddenly leaving off the uses of opium after a long use thereof are great and even intolerable distresses, anxieties and depressions of spirit, which commonly end in a most miserable death, attended with strange agonies, unless men return to the use of opium; which soon raises them again and certainly restores them." Here, Dr. Jones has provided quite a comprehensive description of the symptoms of physical dependence upon a drug. Withdrawal pains following chronic use of opium can be devastating; starting the drug again brings prompt relief. This cycle of dependence is complicated by the fact that with chronic use of the drug, one becomes tolerant and requires progressively larger doses to produce the psychoactive effects.

Scientific insight into the chemical actions of opiates commenced with isolation of the active ingredient. In 1805, a 20-year-old German chemist named

N—CH₃

HO   O   OH

Morphine

N—CH₃

CH₃—C—O   O   O—C—CH₃

Heroin

Chemical structures of morphine and heroin.

Friedrich Sertürner obtained pure morphine from the poppy plant, of which it comprised roughly 10 percent by weight. He named the substance morphine after Morpheus, the Greek god of dreams. Sertürner's isolation of morphine encouraged chemists to seek the active principles of other important medications. Over the next several decades, pure chemicals were obtained from numerous medicinal plants: the active chemicals were isolated from *Digitalis purpurea,* the foxglove plant, and digitalis is still a lifesaving agent in the treatment of heart disease; quinine, the pioneering drug for malaria treatment, was isolated from the bark of the cinchona tree; and cocaine, the first local anesthetic, was extracted from leaves of the coca plant.

As long as medicines were obtained as plant extracts, they could only be administered orally. An advantage of using pure chemicals, such as morphine, is that they can be dissolved in water solutions and injected directly into the bloodstream. This was made possible when Alexander Wood invented the hypodermic syringe in 1853. Analgesia (pain relief without loss of consciousness) was far more reproducible and rapid when the drug was injected than when it was taken by mouth. The first widespread uses of injectable morphine for analgesia occurred in the American Civil War and in the Franco-Prussian War. Indeed, so many Civil War veterans returned home as addicts to injectable morphine that morphine addiction came to be labeled "the soldier's disease."

The twentieth century plague of opiate addiction revolves around the abuse of heroin rather than morphine. Heroin is a fairly simple chemical derivative obtained by adding two acetyl groups to morphine. It enters the brain more quickly than morphine because the acetyl groups increase the drug's ability to dissolve in the brain's fat; one therefore obtains a more rapid "rush" of euphoria following heroin injection. Bayer was the first company to market heroin, introducing it in 1898, two years after the company's introduction of aspirin. Heroin was first offered to the public as a cough medicine, and Bayer promoted it largely on the grounds that it was *nonaddicting*—in contrast to "addicting" cough preparations that, then as now, contained codeine.

The medical profession failed to detect the severe addictive potential of heroin for more than twenty-five years following its synthesis in 1875. As late as 1900 a review concluded, "A sufficiently long period having elapsed since

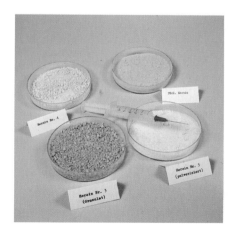

Various forms of pure heroin.

33

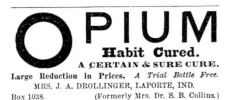

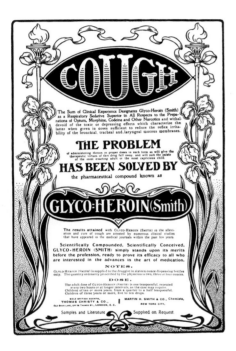

Top Mail-order advertisement published in 1877, aimed at Civil War veterans who had returned home with "soldier's disease." *Bottom* Heroin advertised as a nonaddicting cough remedy.

the introduction of heroin that we are now able to pass judgement upon its real value. . . . Habituation has been noted in a small percentage of cases. . . . However none of the patients suffered in any way from this habituation and none of the symptoms which are so characteristic of chronic morphinism have ever been observed."

The delay in appreciating the dangers of heroin illustrates the impact that mental attitude and physical and social settings can have on whether an addictive drug is abused. Because heroin was introduced as a medicine to treat coughs, patients using it were not seeking or expecting psychoactive effects. Another factor that disguised its addictive potential is that as a cough medication heroin was taken by mouth, considerably slowing the access of the drug to the brain and preventing users from experiencing any sudden euphoria.

How Opiates Act

As noted in Chapter 1, pharmacology is the branch of science that attempts to discover how drugs exert their effects upon the body. At first blush, this might appear to be a fairly uncomplicated task: one has merely to administer the drug to a laboratory animal and measure the drug's effects upon various biochemical systems. However, experience has revealed the many pitfalls of this approach. When such experiments are carried out, scientists usually find that any drug will alter numerous systems in the body, and it is not always possible to distinguish between effects that represent the molecular mechanism of the drug's primary action (the action that brought the drug to the scientist's attention in the first place) and effects that have no connection with that activity. On the other hand, if one has available a series of chemically related agents, some of which are quite potent in eliciting the desired effect while others are inactive and yet others are intermediate, then the problem is less imposing. One can compare the drugs in terms of the extent to which they produce various biochemical effects. With luck, there will be one biochemical action whose relative extent will correlate closely with the relative therapeutic potencies of the various drugs, while for all other effects no such correlation will be observed.

If the experiments work out in this fashion, the researcher can conclude that a particular biochemical action is "associated" with the drug's therapeutic effect; however, this does not prove that the observed biochemical effect is the cause of the clinical one. The correlation could be coincidental, or the associated effect could be a result rather than a cause of the primary action. To better understand this scientific dilemma, consider a scientist from outer space who wishes to discover why some tennis players are better than others. He might begin by obtaining the relative standings of the major tennis players in the world and looking for other variables that correlate with those standings. He would probably find that the size of a player's bank account or the likelihood of a player's owning a Rolls-Royce correlates closely with international rankings, but, of course, this would shed little light upon the factors that make for skill in tennis performance.

The pharmacologists who measured the effect of opiates in the brain on the actions of various neurotransmitters faced just such a dilemma. Their experiments showed the relative pain-relieving effects of different opiates to correlate with changes in *all* of the neurotransmitters. How, then, were scientists to infer which, if any, of the neurotransmitters were causally related to pain relief? Clearly, it would be desirable to locate the initial trigger point where a drug sets off all subsequent metabolic changes that account for pharmacologic effects. When scientists approach the question of drug activity from this direction, they must consider all the known and postulated routes of drug action and focus on those that seem most likely for the drug in question. Some drugs simply diffuse into cells and alter their metabolic machinery directly, though drugs that act in this way are generally not very selective or potent. They require high doses to be effective, and they influence an extremely wide range of body organs. Other drugs initiate their cascade of metabolic changes by binding to a specific protein receptor on the membranes of certain cells in the brain or some other target organ. Binding to such highly specific recognition sites enables these drugs to act very potently and selectively. This seemed a likely mode of action in the case of opiate drugs, some of which are almost unbelievably potent. The opiate etorphine, for example, acts in humans at doses that are a small fraction of a milligram, less than a millionth of an ounce. Such potency is inconceivable unless the drug happens to fit perfectly onto a receptor site that can recognize it at such incredibly minute concentrations. For this reason alone scientists were confident that opiates must act at specific receptor sites.

Another reason for assuming that opiates act at receptors was the existence of opiate antagonists, that is, of drugs that reverse the effects of opiates. Opiates such as heroin kill by depressing the breathing process, and prior to the development of potent opiate antagonists, many victims of heroin overdose died of asphyxiation. Nowadays, patients who overdose can be revived, even from deep and seemingly irreversible comas. Within 30 seconds, intravenous injection of a minute quantity of the opiate antagonist naloxone will completely reverse all opiate effects, rendering the patient alert and apparently normal. Somehow in that short time the naloxone is able to push all the opiate molecules off their receptors.

Antagonists have proven to be as important in brain research as they are in emergency medicine. To explain more fully what a drug antagonist is, however, we must first describe what pharmacologists mean when they speak of an agonist. The name agonist derives from the Greek word meaning "to contend" or "to act": an agonist *acts* at a receptor site to bring about some measurable change in body function. In the case of opiate agonists, such as morphine, the bodily alterations detected are relief of pain and a feeling of euphoria, or well-being. An antagonist may be closely related in chemical structure to the agonist, but it does not produce the same physiological effects. Instead, it selectively and effectively blocks any further agonist activity. As discussed in Chapter 1, the importance of acetylcholine in the memory processes of the cerebral cortex was revealed by the ability of atropine, an acetylcholine antagonist, to disrupt memory. A neurotransmitter called norepinephrine strengthens heart contractions and speeds the rate of beating; conversely, drugs that antagonize norepinephrine are among the most widely used agents in treating angina (a constriction of the arteries in the heart) and high blood pressure.

The chemical differences between opiate agonists and antagonists are generally minor (see the illustration opposite), but when administered to animals or humans, opiate antagonists produce no analgesia and no euphoria. Indeed, many opiate antagonists have essentially no discernible effects in normal subjects. However, opiate antagonists very quickly and thoroughly reverse the effects of opiate agonists. The existence of antagonists in a drug class argues strongly for the presence of specific receptor sites for these drugs. Without receptor recognition sites to compete for, how could an antagonist so selectively block the effects of the agonist?

We have been speaking so far of receptors as if they were nothing more than the recognition sites to which the drug or neurotransmitter molecules become attached. Technically, pharmacologists speak in terms of a "receptor complex" that comprises both the recognition site and the associated second-messenger molecular machinery that translates the recognition of an agonist at the receptor into crucial alterations in cellular activity. Once a drug binds to its receptor site on a neuron in the brain, something must happen so that the neuron fires more rapidly or slowly. Thus, an agonist may be regarded as a drug whose interaction with the receptor brings about a series of events that alter cellular function. An antagonist binds to the same receptor, but without causing any subsequent cellular alterations to take place. Instead, the antagonist merely sits on the receptor, preventing access of other agonist molecules.

Discovering Opiate Receptors

When scientists set out to prove the existence of opiate receptors in the brain, one of the first strategies that occurred to them was to gather evidence that opiates bind to brain preparations hypothesized to contain opiate receptors. The most routine way to do this is to homogenize the brain with a tissue grinder or home blender and centrifuge the tissue suspension at different speeds to obtain neuronal membranes. The membranes can then be mixed with a drug that has been "tagged" with a radioactive tracer. For example, a radioactive form of hydrogen known as tritium can be incorporated into opiate molecules, causing them to give off a radioactive signal. The unbound drug is washed off, and then the tissue is tested for radioactivity. Most biochemical laboratories have machines that can "count" the radioactive emissions and thus measure the amount of drug that has become bound to the membranes.

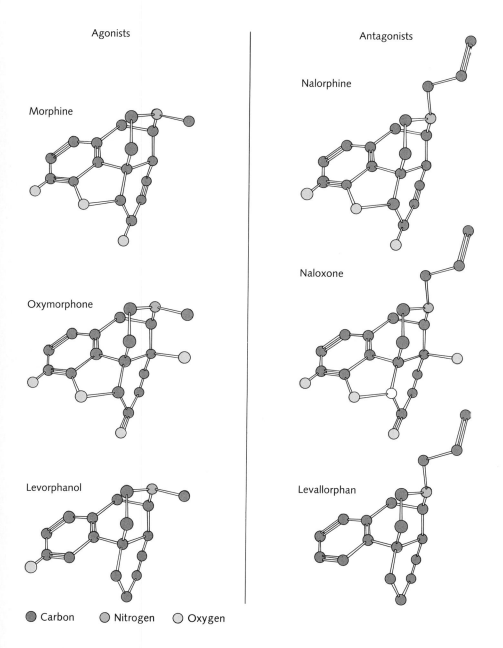

Agonists

Morphine

Oxymorphone

Levorphanol

Antagonists

Nalorphine

Naloxone

Levallorphan

● Carbon   ● Nitrogen   ○ Oxygen

Chemical structures of opiate agonists and antagonists.

Accordingly, as long ago as the mid-1950s, researchers tried mixing radioactive morphine with brain membranes, but their results failed to demonstrate the presence of specific opiate receptors. In these early experiments, the relative strengths with which the drugs bound to the membranes did not parallel their relative pharmacological potencies as opiates. What was the problem?

Scientists readily guessed that these experiments were failing because of the extreme scarcity of opiate receptors in the brain. They knew the typical sizes of clinically effective opiate doses and used them to calculate typical concentrations of the drugs in the brain. The results showed that opiate receptors should constitute no more than one millionth of the brain's weight.

Scientists also knew that while opiates might indeed bind to opiate receptors, they were also likely to interact with a variety of other tissue constituents. Like most chemical compounds, opiate molecules are composed of electrically charged and uncharged portions. Brain membranes contain all sorts of lipids, proteins, and carbohydrates whose positive and negative charges can cause other charged molecules to adhere to them. The membranes also contain uncharged "sticky" surfaces that attract drug molecules by virtue of other chemical properties. Positive charges on the drug would be expected to bind to negative charges on brain membranes, while negative charges on the drug would interact with positive charges on the membrane. Uncharged sticky portions of the drug molecule adhere to sticky areas on brain membranes.

Of course, if there actually were opiate receptors in the brain, researchers expected that opiate molecules would bind more tightly to them than to any nonspecific charged or sticky sites, because opiate receptors, by definition, would constitute a perfect fit for opiate drugs, much like perfectly matched pieces in an erector set. However, if the opiate receptors were as scarce as the data suggested, the number of potential nonspecific binding sites could exceed the number of opiate receptors by a factor of between ten thousand and a million. How could one ever expect to separate the "signal" of an opiate drug binding to its receptor from the vast "noise" of the far more numerous nonspecific binding interactions?

In 1973 Candace Pert and I at Johns Hopkins University, in Baltimore, as well as Lars Terenius in Sweden and Eric Simon in New York, were able to identify the binding of radioactive opiates to receptors in brain membranes and to distinguish specific opiate-receptor interactions from the nonspecific binding of opiates to brain membranes. Our success resulted from some simple but important technical refinements that we made in the radioassay procedure outlined above. First, we took advantage of the fact that opiate receptors can detect and bind very low concentrations of opiate drugs in the receptors' vicinity. The nonspecific binding sites have much less affinity for opiate drugs and so will bind opiates only in the presence of higher opiate concentrations. With this in mind, we decided to use radioactive preparations of the opiate antagonist naloxone that incorporated an extremely high level of radioactivity per naloxone molecule. This permitted us to add minute concentrations of naloxone to the membrane suspension and still obtain enough radioactivity to detect on our counting machines. The low concentrations of naloxone could be expected to bind with far greater preference to opiate receptors than to other nonspecific sites.

In case the highly radioactive naloxone did not by itself suffice to permit detection of opiate receptors, we also employed another technical maneuver: we filtered the brain membrane–naloxone mixture. The great affinity of opiates for their receptors means not only that drugs will bind to them preferentially but also that the drugs will bind more tightly to the receptors than they will to nonspecific binding sites. Accordingly, after incubating the radioactive naloxone with the brain membranes, we poured the membranes and the incubation fluid onto filters, trapping the membranes on the filter material while allowing the incubation fluid with the unbound naloxone to wash away. We even washed the filters several times with water solutions—solutions of salts in water that resemble the composition of body fluids—to remove any naloxone that might still adhere loosely to nonspecific membrane sites. We wanted to remove all naloxone molecules except the ones bound tightly to the opiate receptors. We used a strong vacuum to speed up the filtering procedure, because if we took more than 10 seconds to filter the incubation mixture, the radioactive naloxone would begin to wash off of the opiate receptors as well as off of the nonspecific binding sites.

Using these techniques, we could readily demonstrate specific binding of radioactive naloxone to brain membranes. After that, it was easy to prove that the binding sites we detected were the receptors that account for the pharmacologic effects of these drugs. We simply measured the ability of nonradioactive opiates to compete with radioactive naloxone for the binding sites. The relative potencies of opiates in this competitive process closely paralleled their relative potencies in eliciting opiatelike pharmacological effects. We were even able to show such a parallel in a single tissue (see the illustration on page 42). Opiates inhibit intestinal contractions, an effect that can be monitored in isolated intestinal strips. Potencies of drugs in influencing contractions and in competing for radioactive naloxone binding are closely correlated.

How Receptors Clarify Opiate Effects

With this simple, sensitive, and specific technique for identifying opiate receptors, my colleagues and I at Johns Hopkins could rapidly address a number of important questions. One of the first was the mystery of why agonists differ in their behavior from antagonists, and why antagonists so efficiently reverse the agonist's effects. In initial experiments we found no difference between agonists and antagonists in their affinity for binding to opiate receptors. However, in these first experiments, the brain membranes were immersed in water-based solutions that did not mimic the salt composition of body fluids. All the body's cells are bathed in fairly high concentrations of sodium chloride, as well as other ions, such as potassium, calcium, and magnesium. When Candace Pert, Gavril Pasternak, and I examined the effects of these ions upon receptor activity, we hit pay dirt.

The relative potency with which these drugs bind to opiate receptors in the brain correlates well with their relative abilities to inhibit intestinal contractions.

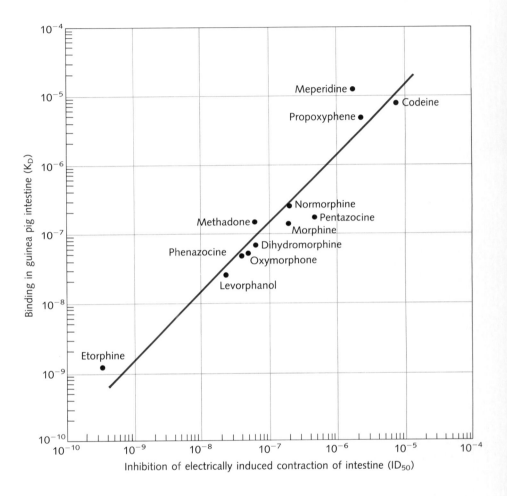

Relatively modest concentrations of sodium ions caused dramatic differences in the behavior of opiate agonists and antagonists. The agonists became much less potent in the presence of sodium, while the antagonists were either not affected or in fact bound better in sodium-containing solutions. Continued research revealed possible reasons for sodium's remarkable effects on receptor binding. In our initial study of opiate-receptor binding, we had focused our attention on the recognition portion of the opiate receptor. Now we speculated that near or adjacent to the recognition site, in the same brain membranes, must be contained the second-messenger machinery that translates the recognition information into changes in cellular function. A variety of evidence suggests that cyclic AMP (see Chapter 1) is the second messenger for opiates; and cyclic AMP levels are regulated by an enzymatic apparatus that is known to

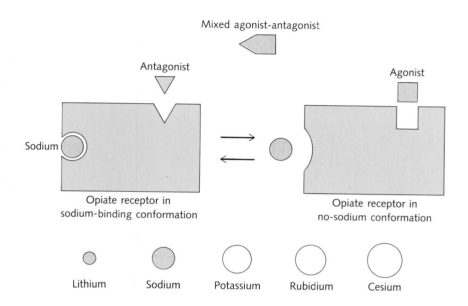

Sodium-binding theory. In this hypothetical model, antagonists bind to sodium-binding form of opiate receptor (*left*), and agonists bind to the non-sodium-binding form. Lithium is the only other positively charged ion to exhibit a similar effect.

use sodium ions. Thus, the effect of sodium upon opiate-receptor binding may reflect an intimate association between the opiate receptor and the cyclic AMP-forming machinery in the neuronal membrane. (See the diagram on page 42.) When agonists bind to the receptor, they bring about key changes in the interactions of sodium with the cyclic AMP apparatus; antagonists do not.

The use of sodium solutions to differentiate opiate agonists from antagonists solved a problem that drug companies had been struggling with since the late 1950s. Around that time they had stumbled upon the existence of opiate drugs that demonstrated both agonistic and antagonistic properties. Unlike naloxone, which is a pure antagonist that does not elicit any of the analgesia and euphoria characteristic of morphine, a number of mixed agonist-antagonist opiates can elicit analgesia but at the same time exercise antagonistic properties that make them less likely to cause addiction. Clearly, this class of drugs offers great promise of providing ideal analgesics: pain relief without addictive potential. Unfortunately, conventional screening tests conducted to identify more such agents failed. We have since learned that while rats treated with morphine and other "pure" agonist opiates do not jump off a hot plate, rats receiving mixed agonist-antagonist opiates do—in fact, they jump as much as rats treated with nothing but saline solution—even though mixed agonist-antagonist drugs effectively control burning pain in humans. Mixed agonist-antagonist opiates were so difficult to identify by experiments in intact animals that by the mid-1970s only a single mixed agonist-antagonist opiate was being marketed, and it was far from ideal since it retained some addicting potential.

When Pert, Pasternak, and I examined the effect of sodium upon the binding affinity of a variety of compounds, we found that opiates fell along a contin-

The sodium ratio compares the drug concentration required to reduce (inhibit) naloxone binding by 50 percent in the presence of sodium to the same concentration in the absence of sodium. It is an accurate predictor of an opiate's agonist, antagonist, or mixed agonist-antagonist activity.

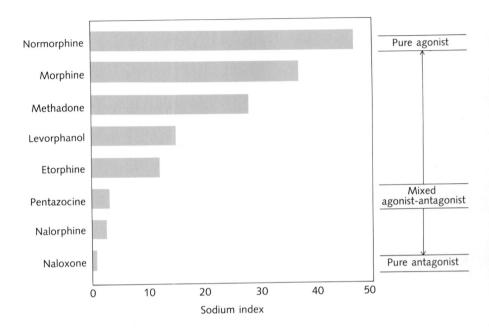

uum. Pure opiate agonists bound much more weakly in the presence of sodium. Pure opiate antagonists were not affected at all. Drugs known to have mixtures of agonistic and antagonistic effects were influenced to an intermediate extent. Thus, monitoring the effects of sodium on opiate-receptor binding provided an efficient means of screening potential mixed agonist-antagonist opiates. One could evaluate fifty drugs in half a day. By contrast, techniques for screening drugs in intact animals generally demand the fulltime attention of a skilled technician in order to evaluate five drugs a week. Not surprisingly, opiate-receptor binding techniques are presently employed routinely in the drug industry.

Locating Opiate Receptors in the Brain

The discovery that opiates do in fact act through specific opiate receptors did not tell us anything about how they relieve pain and bring on feelings of wellbeing. The discovery that receptor interactions trigger alterations in cyclic AMP was similarly unhelpful. Indeed, as of the mid-1970s, although much was known about the biochemical actions of many psychoactive drugs, it was difficult to say just why any of these biochemical effects should produce particular alterations in thinking or feeling. Biochemical experiments in test tubes can never answer such questions, because complex mental functions are mediated by many microscopically discrete brain areas: *where* a neurological activity takes place is as important as *how* it takes place. In the case of opiates, the great breakthrough in understanding came with our ability to identify at a microscopic level exactly which structures in the brain possess opiate receptors.

Although the naked eye can recognize differences in the gross structures of numerous brain subdivisions such as the cerebral cortex and cerebellum, these differences are even more striking when minute brain cell nuclei and neuronal pathways are examined under the microscope. Painstaking neuroanatomical and neurophysiological research conducted throughout the twentieth century had already clarified the apparent functions of many of these microscopic neuronal pathways when, in 1975, Michael Kuhar at Johns Hopkins University developed a technique for viewing neurotransmitter receptors at a microscopic level. Kuhar, Pert, and I applied this technique to the question of opiate receptor localization in hopes that once we knew exactly which neuronal pathways possessed opiate receptors, we might have the key to understanding how opiates affect mental activity. We developed conditions under which certain radioactive opiates, injected intravenously into rats, would concentrate in the nervous system, with virtually all the radioactive drug in the brain bound to opiate receptors. After the rat was killed, very thin brain and spinal cord slices were applied to microscope slides layered with photographic emulsion. It is well known that when radioactive emissions come into contact with a photographic emulsion, they cause the light-sensitive silver grains to record an image. Indeed, Henri Becquerel first recognized the radioactive properties of uranium when a uranium-containing rock in his desk produced a photographic image upon a piece of unexposed film that happened to be sitting next to it. Thus, after exposing the radioactive microscope slides to the photographic emulsion long enough to develop an image, we looked at the slides under the microscope.

The results exceeded our fondest expectations. As you can see in the photographs on page 44, opiate receptors were distributed in very distinct patterns in the brain, with some structures possessing much higher densities than others. What we know of the functions of these structures corresponds nicely with their relative densities of opiate receptors to explain the major pharmacologic effects of opiate drugs (see the table on page 45 and the drawing on page 46). Over the years, neurophysiologists had identified a multitude of brain structures involved in pain perception. Some of the highest densities of opiate receptors were concentrated in areas known to be involved in integrating information about pain.

Pain impulses are usually initiated by trauma to some part of our body surface. This information is transmitted to the spinal cord via long, thin sensory nerves that communicate with various types of spinal cord neurons. Some are long neurons that project up into the brain. Others are small neurons that begin "interpreting" the sensory messages locally by pursuing a dialogue with many other small neurons in a narrow zone in the spinal cord known as the substantia gelatinosa, so called because of its gelatinous appearance. How

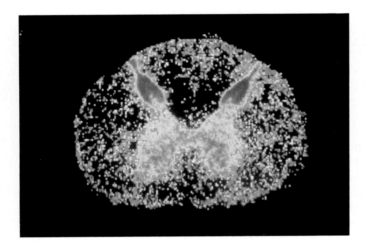
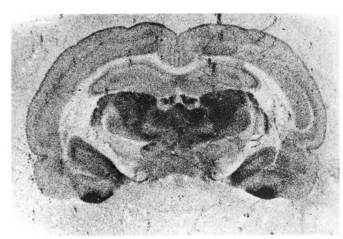

Left Opiate receptors in monkey spinal cord. Highest concentration is in substantia gelatinosa. Orange = highest receptor densities; yellow = low densities; other colors = very low densities. *Right* Distribution of opiate receptors in the brain of a rat. This autoradiogram was produced by adding a radioactive opiate drug to a brain slice. The slice was then exposed to a photographic emulsion, whereupon the bound radioactive drug caused silver grains in the emulsion to "develop" the image you see here.

these neurons integrate information about pain is unclear. Pharmacologists conducting experiments in intact animals had obtained evidence that some pain relief following morphine treatment occurs at the level of the spinal cord. They discovered that morphine has an effect on sensory information processing in the substantia gelatinosa of the spinal cord, where the sensory nerves make their first contacts. We were therefore pleased to note that an extremely dense band of opiate receptors is located in the substantia gelatinosa, accounting for the spinal level of opiate-mediated pain relief.

Opiates relieve pain at the spinal cord level by raising pain thresholds. Thus, if you were treated with morphine, an experimenter would have to administer a more painful stimulus than normal in order for you to notice any pain at all. However, the major analgesic activity of opiates is not so much a raising of the pain threshold as a blunting of the brain's subjective appreciation of pain. Patients who have been treated with morphine because of severe post-operative discomfort or extreme pain from cancer frequently tell their doctors, "It's a funny thing. The pain is still there, but it doesn't bother me." Such changes in conscious responses to pain must be exerted at higher levels in the brain.

Another area with intense concentrations of opiate receptors is the medial portion of the thalamus. The thalamus is the major input portion of the brain; it filters incoming sensory information and sends the most important messages on to the cerebral cortex. The lateral thalamus conveys information about touch and pressure, but the medial thalamus conveys sensory input associated with deep, burning, aching pain—exactly the type that is relieved best by opiate drugs. The table on page 47 compares two types of pain, fast and slow, that are communicated by different classes of nerve fibers. Opiates affect only slow pain.

Localization and possible function of opiate receptors

Location	Functions influenced by opiates
Spinal cord	
Laminae I and II	Pain perception in body
Brainstem	
Substantia gelatinosa of spinal tract of caudal trigeminal	Pain perception in head
Nucleus of solitary tract, nucleus commissuralis, nucleus ambiguus	Vagal reflexes, respiratory depression, cough suppression, orthostatic hypotension, inhibition of gastric secretion
Area postrema	Nausea and vomiting
Locus coeruleus	Euphoria
Habenula-interpeduncular nucleus-fasciculus retroflexus	Limbic, emotional effects, euphoria
Pretectal area (medial and lateral optic nuclei)	Miosis
Superior colliculus	Miosis
Ventral nucleus of lateral geniculate	Miosis
Dorsal, lateral, medial terminal nuclei of accessory optic pathway	Endocrine effects through light modulation
Dorsal cochlear nucleus	Unknown
Parabrachial nucleus	Euphoria in a link to locus coeruleus
Diencephalon	
Infundibulum	ADH secretion
Lateral part of medial thalamic nucleus, internal and external thalamic laminae, intralaminar (centromedian) nuclei, periventricular nucleus of thalamus	Pain perception
Telencephalon	
Amygdala	Emotional effects
Caudate, putamen, globus pallidus, nucleus accumbens	Motor rigidity
Subfornical organ	Hormonal effects
Interstitial nucleus of stria terminalis	Emotional effects

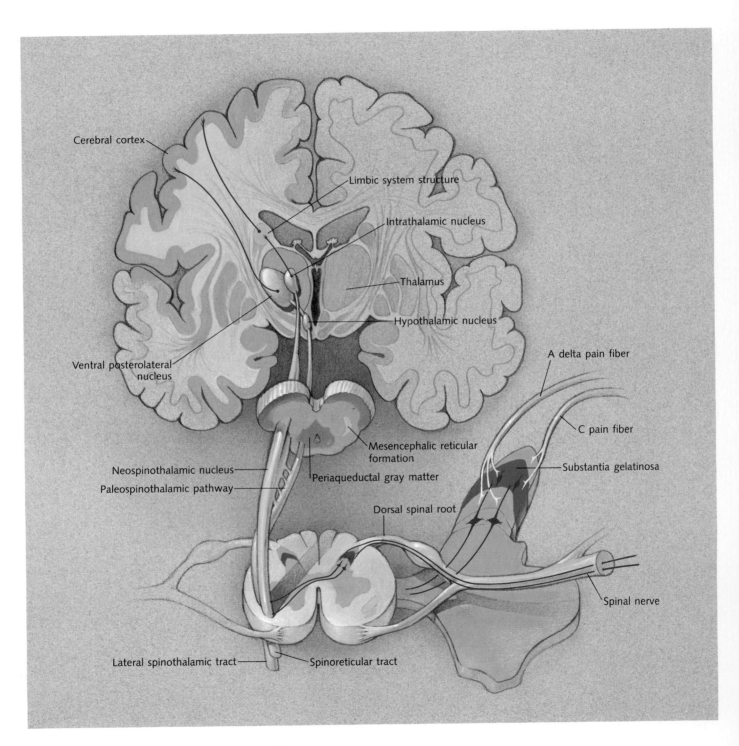

Cerebral cortex

Limbic system structure

Intrathalamic nucleus

Thalamus

Hypothalamic nucleus

A delta pain fiber

C pain fiber

Ventral posterolateral
nucleus

Mesencephalic reticular
formation

Substantia gelatinosa

Neospinothalamic nucleus

Paleospinothalamic pathway

Periaqueductal gray matter

Dorsal spinal root

Spinal nerve

Lateral spinothalamic tract

Spinoreticular tract

Comparison of fast and slow pain

Fast pain	Slow pain
Sharp, pricking	Dull, burning
Group III fibers	Group IV (C) fibers
Short latency	Slower onset
Well localized	Diffuse
Short duration	Long duration
Less emotional overtone	Difficult to endure, emotional autonomic response
Not blocked by morphine	Blocked by morphine
Neospinothalamic system, e.g., dorsal column–medial lemniscus system	Paleospinothalamic system, e.g., medial brain stem and medial thalamus

---

Dense clusters of opiate receptors were also observed in the periaqueductal gray zone of the midbrain, well known to be involved in integrating pain information. Indeed, electrical stimulation in the periaqueductal gray matter produces analgesia.

Even opiate effects unrelated to pain could be explained by the distribution of opiate receptors. For example, opiates constrict the pupils of the eye. This is such a striking effect that police often use it to identify heroin addicts when the persons they suspect are wearing long-sleeved shirts that hide the needle tracks on their arms. The "pinpoint pupils" indicative of a powerful opiate effect are readily apparent. Pupillary diameter is regulated by a variety of structures in the brainstem. Our slides showed that certain of these, the pretectal nuclei, are filled with opiate receptors.

Our slides also explained why excessive doses of opiates kill by depressing respiration. A number of cell groups in the brainstem are involved in regulating breathing or respiratory activity. One of the major areas controlling respiratory reflexes, the nucleus of the solitary tract, has a high concentration of opiate receptors.

Finally, some of the most exciting congregations of opiate receptors may begin to explain how the drugs produce euphoria and, in part, how they initiate the addictive process. Several structures lying just beneath the cerebral cortex are collectively referred to as the limbic system because they form a ring, or "limbus," surrounding the brainstem. A large body of research that began in the 1930s and continues to this day suggests that these structures are the major regulators of emotional behavior.

Facing page Opiate receptors in the nervous system. These receptors are most concentrated in the limbic system, which regulates emotional behavior, as well as in areas such as the medial thalamus and periaqueductal gray, which mediate pain perception.

The limbic system has neuronal connections with many other parts of the brain (see the illustration opposite). For example, neuronal pathways from the limbic system project to the hypothalamus, a part of the brain that is closely linked to the pituitary gland and thereby influences hormone release. These connections enable our emotional state to alter the levels of hormones throughout the body, preparing it in case of a need to fight or flee; they also explain how strong feelings such as anger or grief can influence one's physical health. Because they are closely connected to the cerebral cortex, limbic structures may somehow provide the "feeling tone" that accompanies our thinking processes. For instance, when an idea excites us, our hearts beat faster, our stomachs churn, and we experience a sense of elation, all effects that involve the limbic system. Of the various structures of the limbic system, the amygdala has been implicated most convincingly in originating emotional behaviors and in regulating the hypothalamus and thereby the pituitary gland. A prominent neuronal pathway with cell bodies in the central nucleus of the amygdala sends axons out through a nerve bundle called the stria terminalis to terminate within the hypothalamus.

Other parts of the brain project networks of nerve endings *into* the limbic system. Thus, the locus coeruleus, a small nucleus located in the brainstem, sends its major neuronal projections into the limbic system. The neurons of the locus coeruleus utilize norepinephrine as their neurotransmitter, and norepinephrine is well known to be involved in modulating emotional states.

Various structures in the limbic system collectively contained higher densities of opiate receptors than any other portion of the brain. Particularly striking was the very dense collection of opiate receptors in the amygdala and in the hypothalamus. The locus coeruleus contained an extremely high concentration of opiate receptors. These stood out in striking contrast to the surrounding area of the brainstem, which had far fewer receptors.

The impressive abundance of opiate receptors in the limbic system of the brain suggests a general explanation for the emotional changes caused by opiates, especially for the rush of euphoria brought on by heroin injections. Ideally, we would like to know exactly which structures of the limbic system and which of their connections account for the euphoria. Does one or another portion of the limbic system excite or inhibit certain other structures? Unfortunately, brain researchers do not yet have the means of answering these questions. Emotional behavior is exquisitely subtle and peculiarly human. Animal models of even the simplest types of emotional behavior are difficult to establish, and without an animal model, there is no way to ascertain the role of small individual brain structures in mediating particular behaviors.

Opiate Addiction

The causes of addiction are even more complex than the processes by which opiates influence feelings. Pharmacologists usually consider that addiction has

Facing page Wiring between the limbic system and other parts of the brain. Inputs to the amygdala are traced in red, outputs from the amygdala are shown in white.

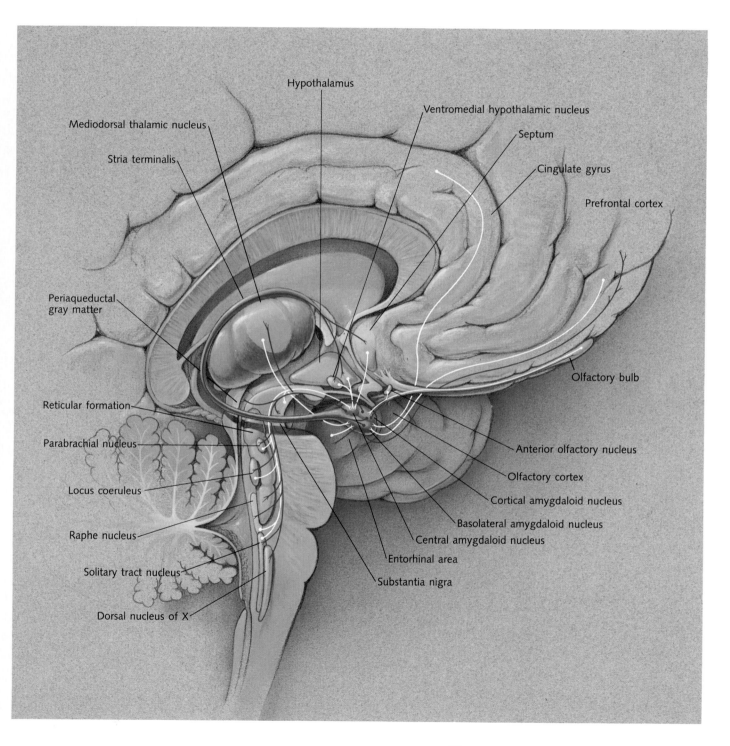

Hypothalamus

Ventromedial hypothalamic nucleus

Septum

Mediodorsal thalamic nucleus

Cingulate gyrus

Stria terminalis

Prefrontal cortex

Periaqueductal
gray matter

Olfactory bulb

Reticular formation

Anterior olfactory nucleus

Parabrachial nucleus

Olfactory cortex

Cortical amygdaloid nucleus

Locus coeruleus

Basolateral amygdaloid nucleus

Central amygdaloid nucleus

Raphe nucleus

Entorhinal area

Solitary tract nucleus

Substantia nigra

Dorsal nucleus of X

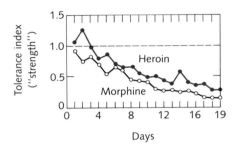

In a study of opiate tolerance, morphine and heroin addicts were given progressively larger drug doses over a period of nineteen days and asked to describe the effects. The tolerance index is the ratio of the dose that would be required by a nontolerant subject to the dose required by a tolerant subject in order for both to experience the same effect.

three components—tolerance, dependence, and compulsive drug-seeking behavior. Tolerance is the first of these to develop following the chronic administration of a drug. It is a condition in which progressively higher doses are required to elicit effects that were at first produced by a very low dose. Tolerance can develop in response to many drugs that are not addicting. One form of tolerance, metabolic tolerance, is a change that takes place in the liver, where drugs are metabolized. Chronic exposure to a drug can stimulate the enzymes in the liver to degrade the drug more rapidly. In other words, the drug effects become shorter-lived because the removal of the drug has been accelerated. People commonly develop metabolic tolerance to aspirin and to penicillin and can also develop metabolic tolerance to opiates. However, the most prominent form of tolerance to opiates and other addictive drugs is called cellular tolerance. People with cellular tolerance have a milder response to a drug even when drug concentrations in the blood and brain are identical to concentrations in someone who has taken the drug for the first time: in cellular tolerance, the brain cells are less responsive than they were when first exposed to the drug.

Physical dependence becomes evident when someone who has chronically ingested a drug suddenly discontinues its use. Severe physical withdrawal symptoms set in, usually opposite in nature to the drug's acute effects. Thus, morphine produces euphoria, somnolence, and relief of pain; when chronic morphine ingestion is abruptly halted, the addicted person becomes overexcited, emotionally depressed, and hypersensitive to painful stimuli.

These first two components of addiction—cellular tolerance and physical dependence—can be readily demonstrated in animals treated chronically with opiates. In contrast, compulsive drug-seeking behavior, the third aspect of addiction, is quite difficult to demonstrate in animals and is thought by some scientists to be a peculiarly human phenomenon. Over the years, thousands of opiate addicts have been arrested on the streets of New York and incarcerated for a year or more in the Federal Narcotics Hospital in Lexington, Kentucky. During this time, they completely withdraw from opiates and have no contact with the drugs at all. In spite of this lengthy abstinence and an extensive program of social and vocational rehabilitation, follow-up usually reveals that discharged patients resume their use of heroin and are again fully addicted in a matter of weeks.

Some scientists feel that compulsive drug-seeking behavior is a sociological phenomenon. These theorists believe that after being discharged from the hospital, the former addicts gravitate back to their old surroundings simply because they do not know any other way of life. Once in their old settings, they almost immediately come into contact with their friendly neighborhood pusher. Other scientists, however, feel that compulsive drug-seeking behavior is biological—that once a person is addicted to opiates, physical changes take place to make him or her forever dependent upon opiates, much as a diabetic is dependent upon insulin. On the basis of current evidence, neither of these two alternative explanations can be ruled out. Similar arguments are advanced in debates about alcoholism. The official position of Alcoholics Anonymous is that alcoholism is a disease whereby the sufferer's brain does not have the capacity to handle alcohol in an appropriate way. Accordingly, the only solution to a drinking problem is total abstention. Even light social drinking will trigger changes that reinstitute the compulsive seeking of alcohol and the full-blown physical addiction.

When we first identified opiate receptors in the brain, Pert and I hoped that we had found a method to solve the riddle of addiction. We speculated that a change in numbers of opiate receptors or in their biochemical properties might explain the addictive process. Unfortunately, after treating rats and mice chronically with morphine for various periods of time and studying the biochemical properties of their opiate receptors in great detail, we were unable to find any alteration that could account for addictive behavior. In the ensuing years, many other researchers have tested opiate receptors for biochemical alterations that could clarify the addictive process, but so far none have been successful.

The Brain's Own Morphine

People are not born with morphine in them. Why then, do opiate receptors exist at all? Using techniques that had successfully identified opiate receptors, neuroscientists went on to identify and analyze receptors for a large number of neurotransmitters. Because the general properties (such as numbers, affinities for drugs, and locations in the brain) of these neurotransmitter receptors were similar to those of opiate receptors, it seemed reasonable to speculate that opiate receptors were designed by nature as receptors for some normally occurring neurotransmitter. Presumably, opiate drugs just happened to fit them nicely. The next step, then, was to search for a normally occurring morphinelike substance.

Two approaches were taken. In Aberdeen, Scotland, John Hughes and Hans Kosterlitz took advantage of the ability of opiates to regulate intestinal contractions. Besides their effects upon the brain, opiates influence the intestine and, in fact, are the most widely used drugs in treating diarrhea. Paregoric, for example, is an alcohol extract, or tincture, of opium, and a typical component of antidiarrheal mixtures. Pharmacologists have for many years monitored the ability of opiates to inhibit electrically induced contractions of intestinal muscle. The fact that this effect is potently and selectively blocked by opiate antagonists such as naloxone suggested that the intestine must have specific opiate receptors (see the diagram on page 53). Hughes and Kosterlitz reasoned that if the brain had an opiatelike neurotransmitter, it should mimic the effects of opiates upon intestinal muscle. They tested many brain extracts and discovered some that did have a morphinelike ability to inhibit intestinal contractions.

51

Principal features of an idealized opiate receptor. The flat surface would accomodate the flat benzene ring of opiate drugs. The anionic (negatively charged) site would bind to the positively charged nitrogen of opiates. Protruding parts of the drug molecules would enter the "cavity" on the receptor surface.

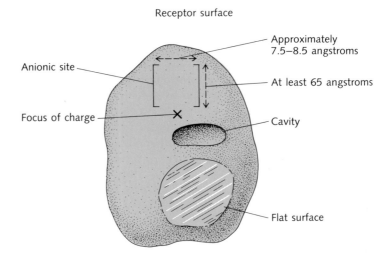

Moreover, the intestinal effects of the morphinelike extracts were potently blocked by naloxone. Hughes and Kosterlitz proceeded to purify the material.

In our own laboratory at Johns Hopkins, Gavril Pasternak, Rabi Simantov, and I used our receptor-binding technology to search for the brain's opiatelike substance. In Uppsala, Sweden, Lars Terenius utilized essentially the same experimental strategy. We added brain extracts to test tubes containing radioactive naloxone and opiate receptors, and we found that certain brain extracts would compete with radioactive naloxone in binding to opiate receptors, just as if the extracts had contained morphine. (By competing with radioactive naloxone, morphine lowers the amount of radioactivity bound to opiate receptors.) The amounts of this opiatelike material in extracts from different brain areas varied in parallel with the variations in numbers of opiate receptors. This convinced us that the brain possessed a normally occurring chemical whose purpose had some connection with the opiate receptor complex.

To separate and purify the various substances, we poured brain extracts through columns of resins. Depending on their ionic charge or molecular weight, various peptides adhered to these resins with more or less avidity. Washing the resins with buffer solutions gradually removed the peptides in accordance with the strength of their adherence. We collected the fluid emerging from the resins in fifty to one hundred test tubes and tested each to see how it competed against radioactive naloxone to bind at opiate receptors.

Hughes and Kosterlitz were the first to successfully isolate and analyze the structure of the opiatelike material. They identified it as a mixture of two small, very similar peptides. (Peptides are chains of amino acids hooked to

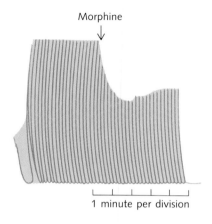

Morphine

1 minute per division

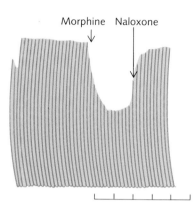

Morphine Naloxone

These polygraph readings show that morphine inhibits electrically induced contractions in guinea pig intestine. Contractions resume after administration of the opiate antagonist naloxone.

each other; proteins are simply very long peptides.) The opiatelike peptides isolated by Hughes and Kosterlitz were extremely short chains, each containing only five amino acids. Four of the amino acids were exactly the same in both peptides, which differed only in the fifth amino acid. The Scottish investigators named these two compounds enkephalins, a term they derived from the Greek for "in the head." A few weeks after Hughes and Kosterlitz published their findings, Rabi Simantov and I completed the chemical identification of the morphinelike material we had been purifying from the brain. It turned out to consist of the same two enkephalin peptides isolated by Hughes and Kosterlitz.

Prior to the isolation of the enkephalins, opiate pharmacologists at scientific meetings had held lengthy discussions about the likely properties of brain extracts with opiatelike activity. A committee had been formed to think of possible names for the substances. The popular choice was endorphins, an abridgement of the phrase *end*ogenous *morphin*elike substances. Hughes and Kosterlitz preferred the name enkephalin, since they reasoned that whatever the substances might be, they would likely have a variety of functions other than their opiatelike activities; the designation endorphin might restrict the curiosity of scientists to the opiatelike effects of the compounds. Since Hughes and Kosterlitz were the first to isolate and identify the structures of these substances, by convention they had the right to name them. However, by the end of 1975, when the enkephalins were isolated, the word endorphin had already been employed extensively by the scientific community and the lay press. Presently, the words enkephalin and endorphin are used interchangeably. Technically, the term endorphin denotes any substance in the body which produces opiatelike effects, while enkephalins are the two specific peptides isolated by Hughes and Kosterlitz. In recent years, other peptides besides the enkephalins have been shown to bind at opiate receptors and to inhibit electri-

Isolation and purification of enkephalins; arrow indicates the enkephalin fraction. The process of purification involved passing brain extracts through columns of beads to which different peptides adhere with different affinities; washing the column with chemical solutions therefore removed different peptides at different rates. Sixty to a hundred fractions were collected into test tubes from each column during the washing process, and the peptide concentration was measured in each. Opiatelike activity was assessed in each fraction by measuring the fraction's ability to compete with radioactive opiates in binding to opiate receptors. With each column, the peak of opiatelike activity could be separated from the bulk of the peptide content, indicating a progressive purification of the opiatelike peptide.

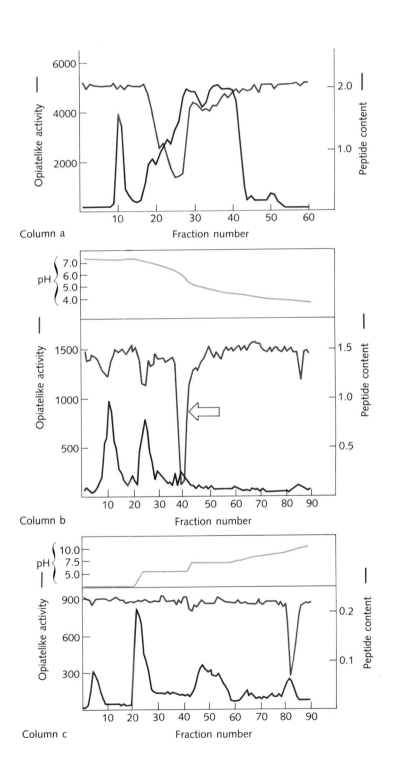

Column a

Column b

Column c

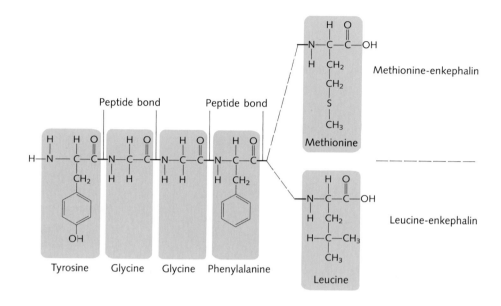

Amino-acid composition of the two enkephalin peptides, which are identical except for the last amino acid in the chain.

cally induced contractions of the intestine. The word endorphin can be used in a generic sense to refer to all of these molecules.

Once the enkephalins were isolated, scores of research projects were launched to investigate their properties. Some important studies used antibody, or immunohistochemical, techniques to identify which neuronal groups in the brain contained enkephalin. First, enkephalin was injected into rabbits or guinea pigs, which in response generated antibodies to remove the foreign substance from their systems. When these antibodies were then applied to thin brain slices on microscope slides, they adhered tightly to enkephalins and to no other substance in the brain. A variety of methods were used either to make the enkephalin antibodies fluoresce or to cause them to develop some type of color that could be recognized under the microscope. This visualization of the antibodies showed researchers where the enkephalin-containing neurons were located.

The resulting pictures provided striking evidence that enkephalins are neurotransmitters. In the first place, they proved that enkephalins are confined to neurons. In the second, by identifying a variety of enkephalin-containing neuronal pathways (see the figure on page 57), they also showed that all enkephalin neurons give rise to dense collections of nerve endings in the same areas as the collections of opiate receptors. Researchers could thus conclude with certainty that enkephalins are the neurotransmitters that normally interact with opiate receptors.

Even before the enkephalins were discovered, neuroscientists had isolated a few peptides that they thought were neurotransmitters. The publicity attend-

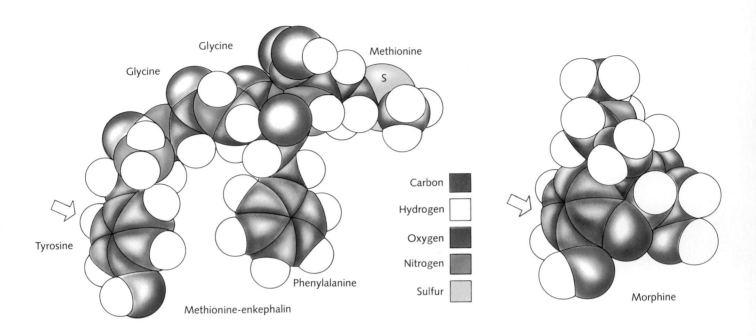

Glycine

Glycine

Methionine

S

Tyrosine

Carbon

Hydrogen

Oxygen

Nitrogen

Sulfur

Phenylalanine

Methionine-enkephalin

Morphine

Comparison of three-dimensional structures of methionine-enkephalin and morphine. Arrows indicate similarities in structure.

Facing page Comparison of opiate and enkephalin receptors in the cervical cord and lower medulla.

ant upon the identification of the enkephalins sparked widespread interest in the possibility that many of the body's peptides act as transmitters. Between 1927 and 1975, fewer than ten neurotransmitters had been described, almost all of a nonpeptide chemical structure. In the next five years, that list grew by about forty definite or probable peptide neurotransmitters: as of 1984, depending on how one evaluates the available data, fifty or more neurotransmitter peptides had been discovered.

Like the enkephalins, most of the other neurotransmitter peptides occupy specific neuronal pathways located in parts of the brain that have important, well-recognized functions. It is therefore more than likely that peptide transmitters play major behavioral roles. Several other peptide transmitters besides the enkephalins are concentrated in the limbic system, where they, too, presumably take part in regulating emotional behavior. One unanswered question is, why did nature create so many different neurotransmitter peptides? Couldn't the brain have made do with a single excitatory and a single inhibitory neurotransmitter? No one yet has the answer, but an army of researchers is looking for clues.

The enkephalins did not escape the notice of the pharmaceutical industry. Drug company researchers were soon wondering whether the enkephalins might be nonaddicting pain relievers. If so, then enkephalin derivatives could prove to be the nonaddicting analgesic drugs pharmacologists had been looking for. Virtually every major drug company in Europe and the United States

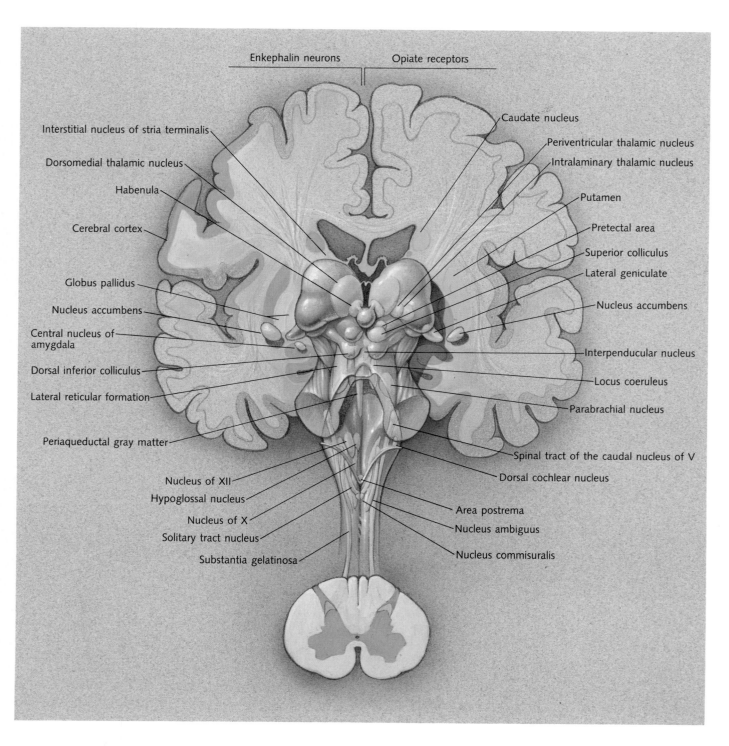

Enkephalin neurons | Opiate receptors

Interstitial nucleus of stria terminalis

Dorsomedial thalamic nucleus

Habenula

Cerebral cortex

Globus pallidus

Nucleus accumbens

Central nucleus of amygdala

Dorsal inferior colliculus

Lateral reticular formation

Periaqueductal gray matter

Nucleus of XII

Hypoglossal nucleus

Nucleus of X

Solitary tract nucleus

Substantia gelatinosa

Caudate nucleus

Periventricular thalamic nucleus

Intralaminary thalamic nucleus

Putamen

Pretectal area

Superior colliculus

Lateral geniculate

Nucleus accumbens

Interpendicular nucleus

Locus coeruleus

Parabrachial nucleus

Spinal tract of the caudal nucleus of V

Dorsal cochlear nucleus

Area postrema

Nucleus ambiguus

Nucleus commisuralis

Enkephalins interact with opiate receptors at the spinal level to suppress pain. Serotonin-containing neurons (5 HT) descend from the midbrain to interact with enkephalin-containing neurons in the substantia gelatinosa. When enkephalins are released, they bind to opiate receptors on substance P-containing pain afferents and inhibit the transmission of pain.

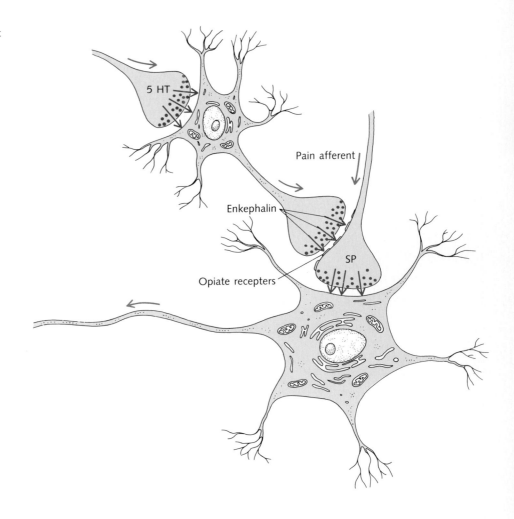

assigned teams to the task of synthesizing and evaluating thousands of chemical derivatives of enkephalin. The first step, well within the range of current pharmacological techniques, was to develop metabolically stable enkephalin derivatives that would not be rapidly destroyed by enzymes in the body. The next task was to tinker with the enkephalin molecules until they could penetrate from the blood into the brain. (We saw in Chapter 1 that electrically charged molecules generally have great difficulty entering the brain.) Although all peptides have both positive and negative charges, chemists were nevertheless able to reduce the molecules' overall charge and thus produce some enkephalin derivatives that could enter the brain to a limited extent. The final step was to alter the derivatives so that they could be absorbed from the stomach into the blood (again, the electrical charges are the problem). This is necessary when a drug is to be administered orally, and it was one of the most difficult aspects of developing a pharmacological enkephalin derivative. Some drug companies have had limited success.

Eventually, out of this vast undertaking by numerous pharmaceutical companies, a consensus began to emerge: enkephalin derivatives certainly can relieve pain, but every compound evaluated has been addicting to a similar extent as morphine. The body's natural enkephalins are not addicting because they are destroyed rapidly by peptide-degrading enzymes as soon as they act at opiate receptors. Therefore, they are never in contact with receptors long enough to promote tolerance and the other changes associated with addiction. In contrast, the qualities that make the enkephalin derivatives stable enough to travel from the stomach to the brain also render them addicting to brain neurons.

As analgesics, the enkephalin derivatives developed by drug companies have not been superior to morphine, or even as good as morphine. Nonetheless, some of them may yet prove to have therapeutic utility. For example, we have seen that the biggest obstacle to developing enkephalin derivatives as analgesics is the fact that their electrical charges make it very difficult for them to be absorbed from the stomach into the blood and from the blood into the brain. This characteristic can probably be used to advantage in the treatment of intestinal disturbances. When paregoric is used to treat diarrhea, the morphine in the mixture passes into the blood, penetrates the blood-brain barrier, and produces its characteristic—and in this case undesirable—effects in the brain. Use of enkephalin derivatives would solve this problem, and several pharmaceutical companies are in fact developing enkephalin derivatives to be used as nonabsorbable antidiarrheal opiates.

In summary, the opiates have proved to be invaluable tools for investigating how the brain perceives pain and regulates our emotional state. The extraordinary success of this field of research has prompted distinguished scientists from many different disciplines to study brain function by utilizing drugs as molecular probes. The story of opiate receptors and enkephalins also serves as a paradigm of how modern molecular techniques can, on the one hand, reveal the ways in which drugs exert their actions on the brain and, on the other hand, furnish strategies for the development of new and better pharmaceutical compounds. In the next chapter, we will see how techniques originally developed to seek out opiate receptors were later used to analyze the effects of antischizophrenic drugs on neuronal transmission in the brain.

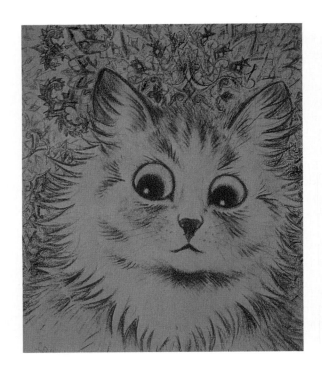

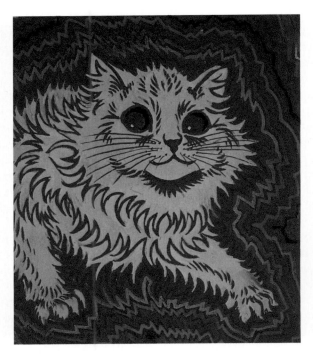

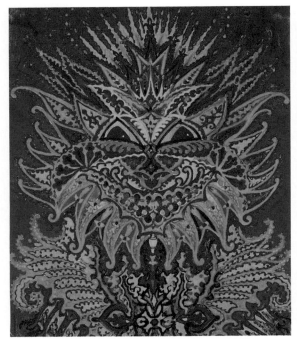

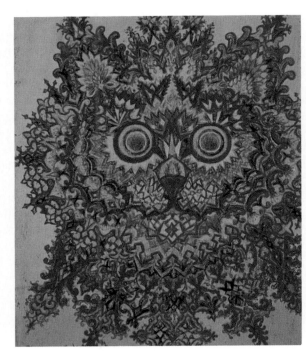

3 | Drugs for Schizophrenia

Among the tools and techniques of modern psychiatry is a large armamentarium of therapeutic drugs. There are drugs that relieve anxiety, others that calm the hyperexcited manic patient, and still others that reverse depressive symptoms. All are valuable, but psychiatrists will generally agree that the most important drugs in the field are those that relieve the symptoms of schizophrenia. Indeed, the development of antischizophrenic, or neuroleptic, drugs represents one of the most important advances in the history of psychiatry.

Calling these drugs "antischizophrenic"—implying that they in some way combat the fundamental schizophrenic process—and proclaiming them to be among the most important developments in psychiatric history are rather strong statements. In this chapter, we will examine the evidence that the drugs do indeed deal with the core of the schizophrenic process. Schizophrenia often lasts a lifetime, the patient is in intense psychic pain, and the loss of earning capacity and the burden on the state exhaust government and social resources, so any drug that can measurably improve the outlook for this most devastating of psychiatric disturbances will obviously be of great importance to psychiatry and to society as a whole. We will begin by exploring the nature of schizophrenia and how these drugs have transformed the lives of schizophrenic patients. Then, we will consider how researchers have attempted to analyze at a molecular level the activity of these drugs in the brain. Insights into this process have greatly enhanced scientists' understanding of the perceptual and cognitive processes that go awry in schizophrenia. Thus, with antischizophrenic drugs, as with opiates, there is a delicate interplay between research whose intent is to clarify the therapeutic actions of the drugs and research that uses the drugs as scalpels to dissect the biochemical underpinnings of mental activity.

Facing page These four paintings are the work of early twentieth century London artist Louis Wain. At the age of 57, Wain began to display symptoms of psychosis. His deteriorating condition is reflected in the progressive disintegration of his cat portraits.

The Nature of Schizophrenia

Schizophrenia is one of the two most common psychotic emotional disturbances. The other, manic-depressive illness, will be examined in Chapter 4. Psychoses are the extremely serious disorders most people think of when they hear the word insane. The psychotic patient is so severely disturbed that he or she loses the ability to interact mentally and emotionally with other people and to assess realistically the meaning and importance of ongoing events. Although anxious or nonpsychotic depressed individuals are often recognized as having irrational fears or disproportionately negative reactions, such people are still generally regarded as being sane. They are still in contact with the environment and make fairly reasonable interpretations of external events. The psychotic person presents a different picture altogether.

The psychosis of schizophrenia is far more devastating to the patients and to everyone around them than any so-called crazy thoughts of a severely depressed but nonpsychotic individual. Schizophrenics may labor under bizarre delusions, totally unrelated to reality. For example, a patient might believe himself to be the Pope and all the hospital nurses to be his bishops. Schizophrenics also experience hallucinations, perceptions of things that are not actually present in the environment. While hallucinations can involve any of the senses—smell, taste, touch, vision, or hearing—schizophrenic hallucinations are usually auditory. Most schizophrenics report hearing voices, usually telling them bad things about themselves: "You are a hideous person with purple skin, and so you must go and shoot yourself." There have been instances in which schizophrenics have committed suicide or murder in obedience to the demands of their "voices."

Although disturbances of perception are often the most dramatic symptoms of schizophrenia, psychiatrists believe that the fundamental abnormalities lie in the schizophrenic patient's thinking processes. Schizophrenics do not think in a logical, cause-and-effect fashion that coincides with events in the real world. Even a fairly conventional or banal conversation with a schizophrenic can leave one feeling that the patient is making mental connections in a loose, tangential, and very vague fashion. The patient's thought processes may be dominated by a powerful conviction that his thoughts are being broadcast to others or that what he is thinking has been "inserted" into his mind by undefined outside sources. In other words, schizophrenics do not feel in control of their own mental processes.

Besides these abnormalities of thought, schizophrenics suffer serious emotional disturbance. Most schizophrenics are withdrawn and fearful of other people, a characteristic psychiatrists refer to as autism. This emotional withdrawal is often designated a "negative" symptom, a term used to describe the absence of healthy behavior, as opposed to "positive," or overtly bizarre, symptoms such as hallucinations and delusions. Some theorists believe that the emotional disturbance, the fear of other human beings, leads the schizophrenic

---

Examples of Schizophrenic Thought Disturbance

These quotations from schizophrenic patients illustrate some of the distorted thinking patterns typical of the disease. They were extracted from *Dementia Praecox or the Group of Schizophrenias*, the classic work in which Eugen Bleuler described the illness and introduced its name.

Thinking and believing opposites at the same time.

> *"She had no handkerchief; she choked with her handkerchief."*
> *"I am Dr. H.; I am not Dr. H."*
> *"I am a human being like yourself even though I am not a human being."*

Blocking of thoughts; the patient's train of thought seems to become paralyzed. Some psychiatrists call this "thought deprivation."

> *"It is as if my mouth was being held closed...as if someone said keep your mouth shut."*

Vague, tangential mental associations.

> *"Dear Mother...I am writing on paper. The pen which I am using is from a factory called 'Perry and Company'. This factory is in England. The city of London is in England. I know this from my school days. Then I always liked geography. My last teacher in that subject was Professor August A. He was a man with black eyes. I also like black eyes. There are also blue and grey eyes and other sorts too. I have heard it said that snakes have green eyes. All people have eyes. There are some too, who are blind."*

---

to separate him- or herself from the rest of the world mentally as well as emotionally—in other words, the emotional disturbance gives rise to the thought disorder. Other psychiatrists believe the thought disorder comes first, that schizophrenics conceptualize the world so differently from others, they are unlikely ever to feel rapport with their fellow beings. Thus the schizophrenic withdraws, and emotional deprivation is the consequence.

Wherever they may stand in relation to this chicken-egg controversy, psychiatrists agree that schizophrenia thoroughly disrupts a person's thinking and feeling. Worse still, in the classic, more serious forms of schizophrenia, the disturbance may persist throughout the patient's life, appearing first in adolescence and progressing gradually from that point on. In the late nineteenth century, the eminent German psychiatrist Emil Kraepelin first identified the diagnostic grouping we now call schizophrenia and labeled it dementia praecox—dementia referring to the mental deterioration, and praecox to its commencement in adolescence or young adulthood. In the early twentieth century, a Swiss psychiatrist named Eugen Bleuler reviewed a large number of case histories and concluded that the thought disorder was fundamental. In other words, Bleuler concluded that the thought disorder appears first and all the

The Proof Is in the Pudding

The following are attempts by schizophrenic patients to interpret some well-known proverbs.

When the cat's away, the mice will play.

"When there's nobody watching, they do things they wouldn't if the cat were there."
"As applied to what? Just gives the mice more liberty."

It never rains but it pours.

"It means nothing more nor less than extremely wet weather."

New brooms sweep clean.

"You can't get in the corners very well with an old broom."
"It means that the quality and also the quantity of any job that can be done with any product is better when new than if it has been used several thousand times."

A rolling stone gathers no moss.

"A moving object is unsuitable for plant growth."
"A stone that keeps rolling doesn't stay long enough to have moss grow on it."
"That a person who is always busy doesn't stop for reflection, doesn't grow in mental and moral stature."

The proof is in the pudding.

"That's my pudding, doctor. All God give forgiveness. Oh, mamma, why did they make expensive weddings? Why don't they stay home, mamma?"
"If you're a good cook, people will like your cooking. The proof is when you eat it."

other symptoms reflect ways in which patients try to cope with their aberrant thinking. He introduced the word schizophrenia to signify the loosening of mental associations apparent in schizophrenic discourse.

While most present-day psychiatrists still agree with Bleuler's definition of schizophrenia (encapsulated in the table on page 65), they frequently disagree among themselves about whether or not a given patient is schizophrenic. To diagnose schizophrenia, the psychiatrist must identify a cluster of symptoms that are hard to define behaviorally and whose genesis is poorly understood. Whether a patient exhibits "loosening of mental associations" is often a matter of opinion. Accordingly, in recent years a set of more specific operational standards for diagnosing schizophrenia has been developed based on the presence or absence of concrete, readily observable behaviors (see the box on page 66). Nevertheless, there are still degrees of uncertainty in the diagnosis of less severe forms of schizophrenia.

Bleuler's classification of schizophrenic symptoms

Fundamental symptoms	Thought disorder
	Blunted affect, indifference
	Withdrawal, retardation
	Autistic behavior and mannerisms
Secondary symptoms, mechanisms patients may develop to cope with the fundamental symptoms	Hallucinations
	Paranoid ideation
	Grandiosity
Nonschizophrenic symptoms, emotional disturbances not uniquely associated with schizophrenia	Anxiety, tension, agitation
	Guilt, depression
	Disorientation
	Somatization (psychosomatic symptoms)

Schizophrenia and Society

One percent of the world's population is affected by classic schizophrenia—schizophrenia in which disturbances are so severe and unmistakeable that virtually all mental health workers will agree in its diagnosis. This is about the same proportion as is affected by diabetes. Another 2 or 3 percent are probably suffering schizophrenic disturbances of lesser severity, without enough textbook symptoms to warrant a hardnosed diagnostic label. Because of the uncertainties noted above, there is considerable debate about the exact incidence of all forms of schizophrenia, and the 2- or 3-percent incidence estimated for only moderately severe schizophrenia has been elevated by some authors to a figure of 5 or 6 percent.

The 1 percent figure for classic schizophrenia has been confirmed by repeated studies conducted in many different countries since the early nineteen hundreds. This incidence is the same in countries to the far north, such as Iceland, and in countries near the equator, such as Brazil. It appears to be the same in democratic and in totalitarian societies, and in times of war and peace, famine and prosperity. This stereotyped invariance in the incidence of severe schizophrenia supports the notion that schizophrenia represents a biologically determined illness.

Strong support for that notion comes from family studies that show children of two schizophrenic parents to have a 40 to 70 percent chance of becoming schizophrenic themselves. Data from studies of twins indicate that this vulnerability is inherited rather than environmental. Identical twins derive from the

Diagnostic Criteria for a Schizophrenic Disorder

This outline is an excerpt from the American Psychiatric Association's *Diagnostic and Statistical Manual–III.*

A. At least one of the following during a phase of the illness:

   (1) bizarre delusions (content is patently absurd and has no possible basis in fact), such as delusions of being controlled, thought broadcasting, thought insertion, or thought withdrawal

   (2) somatic, grandiose, religious, nihilistic, or other delusions without persecutory or jealous content

   (3) delusions with persecutory or jealous content if accompanied by hallucinations of any type

   (4) auditory hallucinations in which either a voice keeps up a running commentary on the individual's behavior or thoughts, or two or more voices converse with each other

   (5) auditory hallucinations on several occasions with content of more than two words, having no apparent relation to depression or elation

   (6) incoherence, marked loosening of associations, markedly illogical thinking, or marked poverty of content of speech if associated with at least one of the following:

      (a) blunted, flat, or inappropriate affect

      (b) delusions or hallucinations

      (c) catatonic or other grossly disorganized behavior

B. Deterioration from a previous level of functioning in such areas as work, social relations, and self-care.

C. Duration: Continuous signs of the illness for at least six months at some time during the person's life, with some signs of the illness at present. The six-month period must include an active phase during which there were symptoms from A, with or without a prodromal or residual phase, as defined below.

Prodromal phase: A clear deterioration in functioning before the active phase of the illness not due to a disturbance in mood or to a Substance Use Disorder and involving at least *two* of the symptoms noted below.

Residual phase: Persistence, following the active phase of the illness, of at least *two* of the symptoms noted below, not due to a disturbance in mood or to a Substance Use Disorder.

Prodromal or Residual Symptoms

   (1) social isolation or withdrawal

   (2) marked impairment in role functioning as wage-earner, student, or homemaker

(3) markedly peculiar behavior (e.g., collecting garbage, talking to self in public, or hoarding food)

(4) marked impairment in personal hygiene and grooming

(5) blunted, flat, or inappropriate affect

(6) digressive, vague, overelaborate, circumstantial, or metaphorical speech

(7) odd or bizarre ideation, or magical thinking, e.g., superstitiousness, clairvoyance, telepathy, "sixth sense," "others can feel my feelings," overvalued ideas, ideas of reference

(8) unusual perceptual experiences, e.g., recurrent illusions, sensing the presence of a force or person not actually present

Examples: Six months of prodromal symptoms with one week of symptoms from A; no prodromal symptoms with six months of symptoms from A; no prodromal symptoms with two weeks of symptoms from A and six months of residual symptoms; six months of symptoms from A, apparently followed by several years of complete remission, with one week of symptoms in A in current episode.

D. The full depressive or manic syndrome (criteria A and B of major depressive or manic episode), if present, developed after any psychotic symptoms, or was brief in duration relative to the duration of the psychotic symptoms in A.

E. Onset of prodromal or active phase of the illness before age 45.

F. Not due to any Organic Mental Disorder or Mental Retardation.

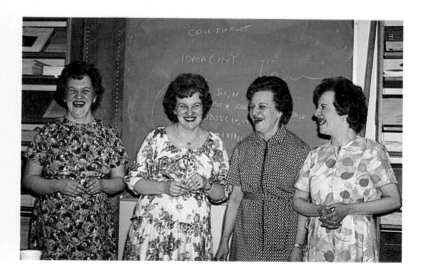

The Genain sisters are identical quadruplets, all diagnosed as schizophrenic. Their case provided psychiatrists with a remarkable study in the disease's etiology, for though these women share identical genes, each exhibits a different degree of illness.

67

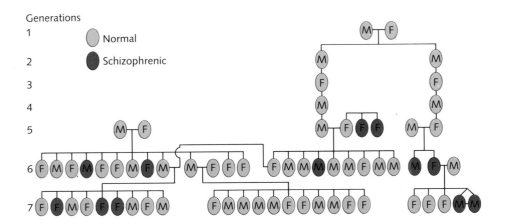

Generations

1 ○ Normal

2 ● Schizophrenic

This genogram, or family tree, diagrams a high incidence of schizophrenia in two Swedish families joined by marriage. Twelve of the sixty-eight individuals represented here were afflicted with schizophrenia, an incidence nearly eighteen times greater than normal.

same fertilized egg and have identical genes, while fraternal twins have no greater genetic similarity than conventional siblings. Of course, whether or not their genes are identical, twins are generally raised in the same family, with the same childhood surroundings and mode of upbringing. It is interesting then that if one of a pair of identical twins becomes schizophrenic, studies show a greater than 50 percent probability that the other twin will develop the disease as well, while, in contrast, the concordance rate for fraternal twins—that is, the rate at which the fraternal twins will "concord" with each other in developing schizophrenia—is only 10 or 15 percent.

Research on the genetics of schizophrenia has yielded many insights into the relative roles of "nature" and "nurture" in the development of schizophrenic behavior. If schizophrenia were fully determined by genetic factors, the concordance rate in identical twins would be 100 percent, yet in about 50 percent of cases where one identical twin is schizophrenic, the other twin seems fairly normal. Many researchers have sought to identify environmental factors that might contribute to the development of schizophrenia in one twin while sparing the other. Several studies have indicated that the twin destined to become schizophrenic weighed less at birth and had more physical disability during the first few days of life than the co-twin who did not become schizophrenic. Thus, it would appear that the most readily delineated "environmental" factor predisposing to schizophrenia is not the psychological environment but the uterine environment.

Discovering the cause or causes of schizophrenia is of the gravest importance, for the impact of the disorder on the overall health of the nation is grossly out of proportion to its statistical incidence. Up until the early 1950s, a large segment of the country's schizophrenic population lived in state mental hospitals from which many of them never emerged; and because conditions in

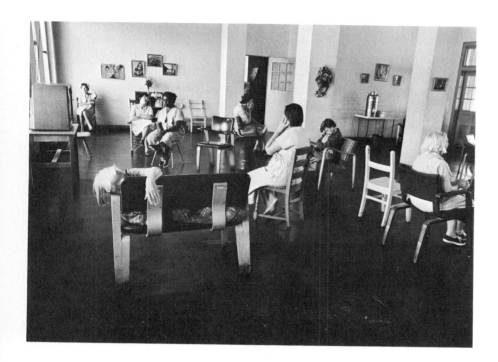

Contrasts between mental hospitals. The scene in the upper photograph demonstrates some attempt on the part of the institution to create a pleasant atmosphere that fosters patients' strengths. The facility shown below seems impersonal, isolating, and even punitive.

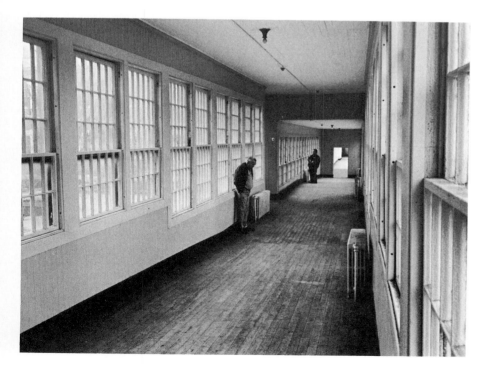

those hospitals were likely to be inferior to the conditions in bad prisons, a diagnosis of schizophrenia was, in effect, a sentence to a living death. Patients who managed to stay out of the hospital were greatly disabled by their disease and usually unable to work, and the cost to society in loss of productivity and in government support for such people was astronomic.

Records show that in 1955 one out of every two hospital beds in the United States was occupied by a psychiatric patient. Half or more of these patients were schizophrenic, while the remainder represented an assortment of physical and social disabilities such as alcoholism, cerebral arteriosclerosis, and destitution in old age. These numbers, while disturbing, are easily explained. A patient with heart disease, cancer, or diabetes might be hospitalized on three or four occasions for a couple of weeks each time. A patient diagnosed as schizophrenic in the 1950s might stay hospitalized for 50 years.

The Impact of the Neuroleptic Drugs

Chlorpromazine, the prototype neuroleptic agent, entered European psychiatric practice in 1952 and was introduced in the United States in 1955. It met with immediate acceptance by the staffs of large mental hospitals both in Europe and North America, and it improved patient behavior so dramatically that before long virtually every hospitalized schizophrenic was being treated with the drug. Soon after chlorpromazine was introduced in the United States, the population of the state mental hospitals—which until then had been increasing by 10 or 15 percent yearly—began to plummet. Today, in 1986, the state mental hospital population is only a third of what it was thirty years ago. Considering population trends in the country as a whole, without neuroleptics our mental hospitals would now be housing ten times the number of patients that actually occupy them today.

Some researchers argue that the introduction of chlorpromazine and the simultaneous decline in the population of state hospitals are coincidental. These researchers believe that much of the decline in the hospitalized patient population can be attributed to the community mental health movement that gained momentum toward the end of the Eisenhower administration, when community mental health centers were introduced throughout the country. The purpose of these centers was to treat mental patients close to home rather than in faraway, impersonal state institutions. Proponents argued that it would be easier to restore the mentally ill to a functional status in society if they could remain with family and friends during the course of their treatment. This system of therapy and rehabilitation has done much for the plight of all emotionally disturbed people; however, it would not have been as readily developed but for the simultaneous introduction of neuroleptic drugs, with their ability to reduce the intensity of even the severest symptoms to a level at which they can be managed outside of locked wards.

In itself, the deinstitutionalization of large numbers of schizophrenic patients has provoked much controversy. Many people are appalled at the large numbers of individuals wandering the streets of big cities obviously mentally disturbed and seemingly unable to care for themselves. While the problem is largely sociological and political, a result of state and federal governments' efforts to reduce the cost of caring for the mentally ill, it does dramatically illustrate the limitations of neuroleptic drugs. Neuroleptics may be uniquely and selectively effective in alleviating the severity of schizophrenic symptoms, but they do not actually cure the disease. Moreover, even after long-term treatment with high doses, many schizophrenic patients continue to exhibit substantial mental disturbance. Perhaps that is why, after years of established use, some psychiatrists still question whether neuroleptics actually do anything special. This debate has an interesting history.

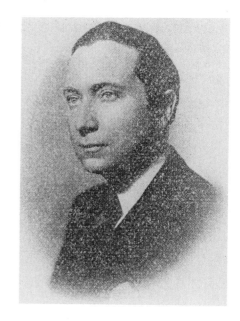

The Discovery of the Neuroleptic Drugs

As with so many drugs in medicine, the discovery of the first antischizophrenic agent was a combination of accident and good judgment. It happened in 1950, when the French neurosurgeon Henri Laborit was attempting to prepare a cocktail of various medications to give to patients prior to instituting anesthesia. His aim was to quiet the patients and relieve their fears before putting them to sleep. He also hoped his concoction would protect the patient's body from the dangers that anesthesia can pose to the heart and other organs.

Laborit had a theory that histamine released during anesthesia accounted for many sudden deaths. Accordingly, he asked the Rhone-Poulenc Drug Company to supply him with a compound called promethazine, an antihistamine that was known to be fairly sedating. After testing promethazine, Laborit was so pleased with the results that he asked the company to send him any drugs they had that were related to promethazine. One of these, chlorpromazine, had originally been developed as a potential antihistamine, but the company considered it too sedating and not a strong enough antihistamine. Laborit, however, was so enthusiastic about the "beatific quietude" that chlorpromazine elicited in his surgical patients that he recommended the drug to his psychiatrist colleagues for use in calming agitated patients.

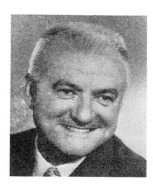

Jean Delay (1907–   ) (*top*) and Pierre Deniker (1917–   ), the French psychiatrists whose use of chlorpromazine in escalated doses led eventually to a general appreciation of the drug's antischizophrenic properties.

Most of the psychiatrists who tried low doses of chlorpromazine on their patients did not find it to be effective. Fortunately, two Parisian psychiatrists, Jean Delay and Pierre Deniker, seem to have been unaware of their colleagues' negative results. In 1951, Delay and Deniker began to administer chlorpromazine to their patients in progressively increasing doses, eventually reaching levels substantially higher than those prescribed by their colleagues. With these escalated doses, they began to see clear-cut improvement, and in a surprising variety of patients. Agitated, anxious patients, hyperactive manics, and schizophrenics all became more manageable.

Although the success witnessed by Delay and Deniker seemed to stem from the sedating effects of the drug, chlorpromazine differed dramatically from classic sedatives, such as barbiturates, in that it did not put patients to sleep, even at fairly high doses. Instead, the drug performed a special role in the treatment of insanity by making difficult patients more manageable without rendering them unconscious. As time passed and psychiatrists acquired experience with chlorpromazine, many of them began to feel that the drug had an even more remarkable ability, quite apart from its special efficacy as a sedative.

Are Neuroleptics Antischizophrenic?

When psychiatrists refer to neuroleptics as antischizophrenic drugs, they are implying that these drugs alter, temporarily, some fundamental schizophrenic abnormality in the brain. The suggestion is that neuroleptics are more than simple mental straitjackets for calming hyperactive patients and allowing them to be managed outside of hospital walls. The distinction is crucial, for if the drugs are truly antischizophrenic and scientists can understand how they act in the brain, the knowledge might shed light on what is aberrant in schizophrenia. As we discussed above, family studies have revealed a major genetic component in the development of schizophrenia. Genetic abnormalities imply specific molecular abnormalities. In fact, it is conceivable that a single biochemical alteration is at the root of schizophrenia. Neuroleptic drugs, if truly "antischizophrenic," could be used to probe the biochemistry of the brain and find the site of this abnormality.

Delay and Deniker came to believe that chlorpromazine influenced schizophrenic patients in a unique fashion that could not be explained as a simple calming effect. The two psychiatrists were convinced that the "craziness" itself was being lessened, and in so selective a way that they suspected the drugs were acting at some specific location in the brain. They had noticed that when they gave the drug to schizophrenic patients, the first appearance of improvement was accompanied by symptoms reminiscent of Parkinson's disease. This is a neurological disease of unknown cause that primarily affects motor functions, causing rigidity, difficulty in moving, and a tremor of the limbs. The persistent association of these neurological side effects with the improvement in schizophrenic symptoms was in fact the reason Delay and Deniker called the drugs neuroleptic, a term they derived from the Greek, meaning "to clasp the neuron."

Subsequent events helped to determine whether chlorpromazine acted directly upon the schizophrenic thought disorder or merely calmed the patient's agitation so that the thought disorder could fade away of itself. For one thing, the success of chlorpromazine prompted drug companies to synthesize literally thousands of derivatives. Some of these chemical relatives of chlorpromazine were not sedating at all, and yet relieved schizophrenic symptoms just as well as chlorpromazine did. For another, while chlorpromazine calmed hyperactive schizophrenics, it was also reported to have the additional and complementary virtue of "activating" schizophrenics who were withdrawn. If the drug were acting only as a sedative, it should cause patients who are already underactive to deteriorate further.

Psychological investigations, too, were confronting the antischizophrenic issue. In some studies, each component of a patient's thinking and feeling was evaluated separately from the rest, and for every component the effects of neuroleptic drugs were compared with those of an inactive placebo and also with those of comparably sedating doses of nonneuroleptics, such as barbiturates. Neuroleptics and barbiturates showed the same ability to relieve anxiety and agitation, but neuroleptics clearly diminished the thinking disturbance of schizophrenics, whereas barbiturates were no better than placebos.

Taken as a whole, the preponderance of evidence seems to favor the notion that neuroleptics are indeed antischizophrenic drugs. Accordingly, knowing their site of action in the brain should have major implications for an understanding of schizophrenia.

Clues from Reserpine

In attempting to unravel how a drug exerts its therapeutic action, the pharmacologist makes use of every glimmer of evidence. One early and very fruitful clue lay in Delay and Deniker's observations that schizophrenic patients who took chlorpromazine began to improve at about the same time that the drug began to induce Parkinsonian side effects. The association was so striking that their published "cookbook" for treating schizophrenics instructed physicians to administer progressively increasing doses without stopping until Parkinsonian symptoms such as muscular rigidity, weakness, and tremor were in evidence.

These clinical observations led Delay and Deniker to suggest that chlorpromazine might have one primary biochemical effect. In one part of the brain this effect would cause symptoms resembling Parkinson's disease; in another brain region, the same chemical effect would relieve schizophrenic symptoms. Researchers using a drug called reserpine soon obtained clinical results that supported this idea.

Today, reserpine is used primarily to treat high blood pressure. It is the active ingredient extracted from the Indian snakeroot plant, which had been used in Indian folk medicine as a treatment for many conditions. In 1931, Indian physicians established the effectiveness of snakeroot, whose botanical name is *Rauwolfia serpentina*, in relieving high blood pressure. Some twenty years later, chemists at the Ciba Drug Company isolated reserpine from the plant and commenced clinical studies of its effects in hypertension. Its efficacy was so striking that, despite the subsequent introduction of scores of other antihypertensive agents, reserpine is still one of the mainstays in controlling high blood pressure.

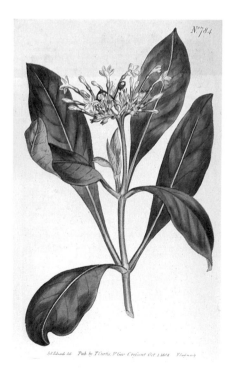

Rauwolfia serpentina, or snakeroot, the natural source of reserpine.

73

One traditional use of the *Rauwolfia* plant was in the treatment of mental patients. The American psychiatrist Nathan Kline initiated studies of the effects of reserpine on schizophrenics at just about the time that Delay and Deniker were investigating chlorpromazine. Kline reported remarkably effective relief of schizophrenic symptoms with reserpine, and a clinical response quite similar to that obtained with chlorpromazine. Considering that the two drugs differed greatly in their chemical structure (illustrated opposite), these were most intriguing results.

The similarity between the actions of reserpine and chlorpromazine carried over into their side effects. Reserpine, too, produced Parkinsonian symptoms. Moreover, as with chlorpromazine, these side effects usually began with doses just high enough to alleviate schizophrenic disturbances.

Here was a clue of great value. Two very different chemicals produced almost identical clinical pictures. First, it meant that a single biochemical event might well account for both the Parkinsonian side effects and the therapeutic antischizophrenic actions. Second, it simplified the task of research pharmacologists in working out the molecular mechanism of pharmacological activity—*two* drugs, with different structures but similar clinical profiles, were now available for study. Correlation experiments were now possible. Pharmacologists could administer the drugs to rats and then test the rats for biochemical alterations. If they found that reserpine caused ten chemical changes, only one of which was also exerted by chlorpromazine, then the chemical change elicited by both drugs would most likely represent the molecular mechanism of therapeutic activity.

Dopamine in Parkinsonism

Just about the time that chlorpromazine and reserpine were being introduced to psychiatry, a revolution in the understanding of brain chemistry was taking place. In the middle to late 1950s, techniques were developed enabling scientists to measure the amounts of certain biogenic amines in the brain, and evidence was building that the substances were, in fact, major neurotransmitters. Biogenic amines, illustrated on page 76, are naturally occurring, or "biogenic," compounds that contain an amine structure, that is, a nitrogen linked to hydrogens or carbons. The best-known biogenic amines are dopamine, norepinephrine, and serotonin.

In 1955, Parkhurst Shore and Bernard Brodie at the National Institutes of Health in Bethesda, Maryland, administered reserpine to rats and then measured the levels of serotonin in the rats' brains. They were amazed to find that reserpine treatment virtually depleted the brains of their serotonin content. Subsequently, other scientists found that reserpine similarly depletes the brain of norepinephrine. Dopamine was first demonstrated to exist in the brain in 1958, and soon thereafter researchers found that reserpine also depleted the brain of its dopamine.

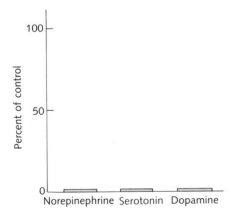

In a typical experiment to determine the effects of reserpine on brain amines, rats are injected subcutaneously with 1 milligram per kilogram of reserpine. Levels of norepinephrine, serotonin, and dopamine are all close to zero.

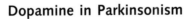

Chlorpromazine

Reserpine

The latter results immediately explained the Parkinsonian effects of reserpine. Neuropathologists had known for many years that classical Parkinson's disease is associated with abnormalities in a group of brain structures called the corpus striatum, a part of the brain well known to regulate motor behaviors. When dopamine was originally measured in the brain, scientists noticed that it was very highly concentrated in the corpus striatum, with much lower levels in other brain regions. By contrast, the corpus striatum possesses relatively little norepinephrine or serotonin. Accordingly, scientists speculated that reserpine produced symptoms mimicking Parkinson's disease by depleting the corpus striatum of its dopamine content.

In Vienna in 1960 the pharmacologist Oleh Hornykiewicz tested this hypothesis by measuring dopamine in the brains of patients dying with Parkinson's disease. He found that dopamine levels in the corpora striata of many patients with Parkinson's disease were only 20 percent of normal, while the levels of other chemicals in the same region were well within normal parameters. The condition of the Parkinsonian patients resembled that of the rats treated with reserpine, but with one big difference: while reserpine depletes the brain of all three biogenic amines, patients with Parkinson's disease showed pronounced abnormalities in dopamine levels alone. There was some loss of norepinephrine in the brain, but this was minor compared to the massive depletion of dopamine.

To sum up, by 1960 several clues linked dopamine levels in the brain with the Parkinsonian side effects of reserpine. Reserpine depleted dopamine, norepinephrine, and serotonin, but only dopamine was deficient in Parkinsonism. Moreover, since all neuroleptics elicited the same clinical effects as reserpine, it seemed logical to infer that they all caused the same or similar chemical changes in the brain.

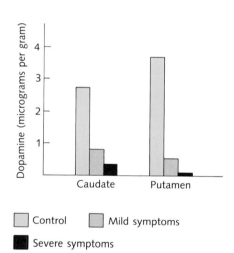

Control   Mild symptoms

Severe symptoms

These data from the research of Oleh Hornykiewicz and associates show the profound depletion of dopamine from the two major parts of the corpus striatum in patients afflicted with Parkinsonism. The severity of symptoms correlates with the amount of dopamine depletion, which in turn reflects the degeneration of the dopamine-containing neurons. Levels of most other neurotransmitters in Parkinsonian brains were found to be normal or much closer to normal than were dopamine levels.

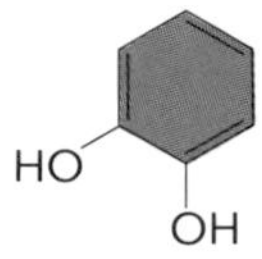

Catechol

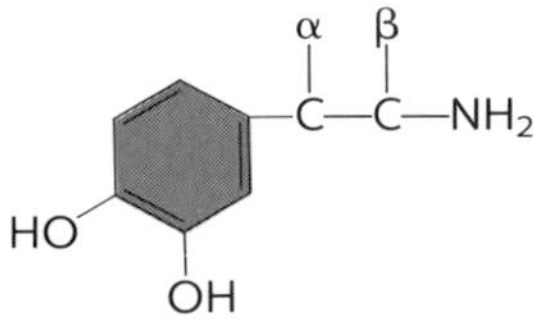

Catecholamine

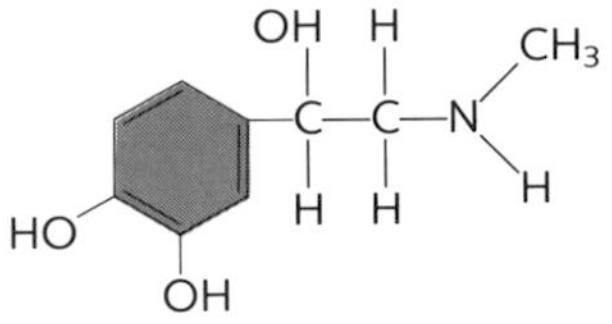

Epinephrine

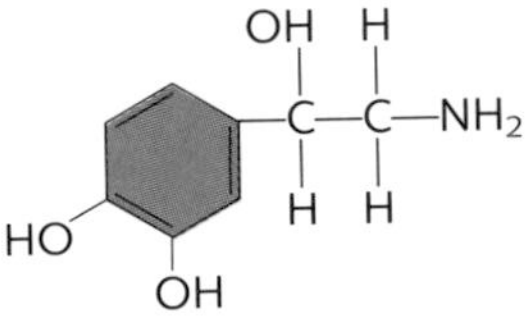

Norepinephrine

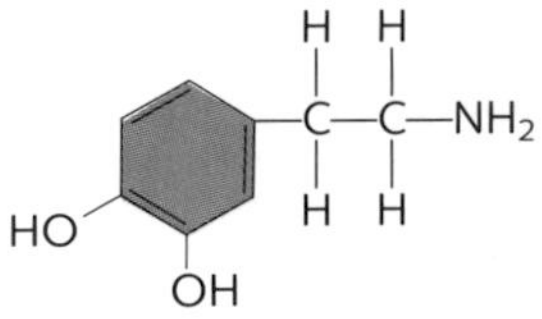

Dopamine

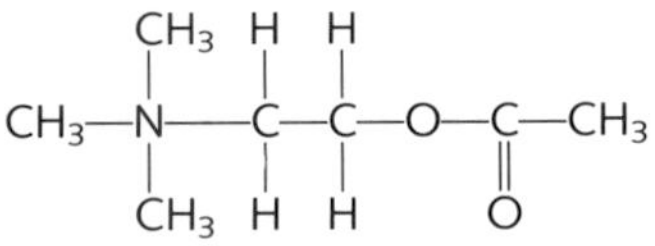

Acetylcholine

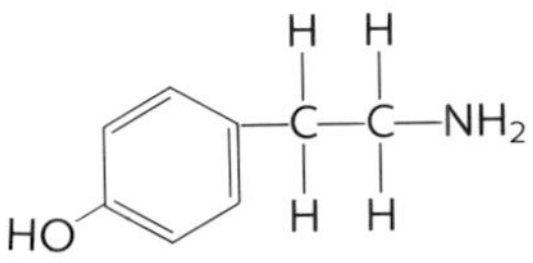

Tyramine

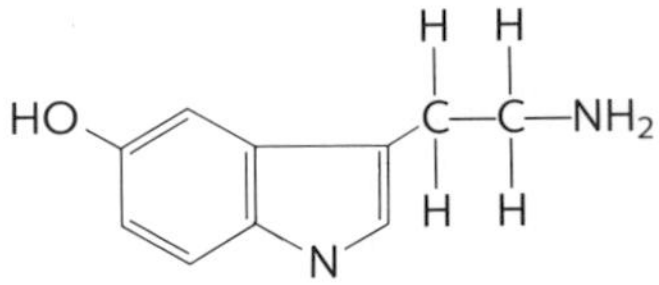

Serotonin (5-hydroxytryptamine)

Chemical structures of a number of biogenic amines. General features of these molecules are their small size and positively charged nitrogen atom. Epinephrine, norepinephrine, and dopamine all contain a catechol moiety and are therefore designated catecholamines.

Neuroleptics and Dopamine Receptors

Considering the similarities in clinical effects of reserpine and chlorpromazine, the Swedish pharmacologist Arvid Carlsson assumed that treating rats with chlorpromazine would cause their brains to be depleted of norepinephrine, serotonin, and dopamine. However, when he tested this assumption, he was surprised to find completely normal levels of all three neurotransmitters. While he might have concluded at this point that the "dopamine theory" was wrong, Carlsson instead took an alternate approach to testing the effects of neuroleptics on dopamine. First of all, he was not restricted to the use of chlorpromazine. Numerous neuroleptic drugs were available that varied greatly in their antischizophrenic potencies. They also varied, in a parallel fashion, in the severity of their Parkinsonian side effects. Carlsson expected that the particular biochemical effect responsible for the antischizophrenic actions of neuroleptics would also vary from drug to drug in parallel with their clinical potencies. In other words, if one drug were one hundred times more potent than a second drug in eliciting a particular biochemical response, but the second drug was a more potent antischizophrenic agent, one could rule out that particular biochemical response as the mediator of the therapeutic effect. A perfect correlation between biochemical response and therapeutic action in a series of thirty drugs would be even more revealing.

Second, Carlsson was not restricted to measuring levels of the neurotransmitters themselves. He was also able to measure concentrations of their metabolites, or breakdown products. In the course of cell metabolism, all chemicals in the body are broken down to simpler products that are either recycled for repeated use or eliminated from the system as waste. Sometimes levels of metabolites tell us more about the disposition of the parent compound than levels of the parent compound itself. For example, metabolites provide hints about the firing rates of neurotransmitter-containing neurons. If a neuron fires more rapidly, it releases more neurotransmitter molecules, which are in turn broken down into higher-than-normal concentrations of neurotransmitter metabolites. Levels of a neurotransmitter itself do not necessarily fall in these circumstances, because the neuronal machinery that synthesizes the neurotransmitter accelerates to accommodate the speeded up firing rate. This ability of the neuron ensures that it will not run out of transmitter molecules when the demand for transmitters is increased. Thus, if brain tissue is found to contain more metabolites than normal, one can infer that the neurons have been firing more rapidly (see the figure on this page).

When Carlsson administered a series of different neuroleptics to rats, he did find changes in the levels of metabolites for norepinephrine and dopamine even though levels of the transmitters themselves were unchanged. Some neuroleptics caused elevation of metabolites of both norepinephrine and dopamine. Other neuroleptics elevated only one type of metabolite or the other. The final results showed that relative increases in dopamine metabolite levels by different neuroleptics paralleled the relative clinical potencies of the neuroleptics. By contrast, relative potencies of neuroleptics in increasing norepinephrine metabolites had no relationship with the relative clinical potencies of the drugs. In other words, a phenothiazine such as promethazine, which is not antischizophrenic at all, increased norepinephrine levels as much as did haloperidol, an extremely effective and potent antischizophrenic drug. The inescapable conclusion was that higher levels of norepinephrine metabolites had no relation to the clinical actions of neuroleptics in relieving schizophrenic symptoms, whereas there did seem to be such a relationship with dopamine metabolites. Increased levels of dopamine metabolites reflect increased firing rates of dopamine neurons, and it appeared that the more potent a drug was in accelerating the firing of dopamine neurons, the more potent a neuroleptic it was in relieving schizophrenic symptoms.

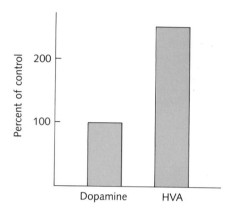

In a typical experiment to compare the effect of chlorpromazine on brain dopamine and on homovanillic acid (HVA), a dopamine metabolite, rats are injected intramuscularly with 15 milligrams per kilogram of chlorpromazine. Six hours later, the rats are killed and their brains are tested for dopamine and HVA. The drug increases HVA levels, although dopamine levels remain unchanged.

An increase in the level of dopamine break-down products may indicate that dopamine neurons are firing more rapidly. The mechanism of dopamine breakdown metabolism speeds up in response to the presence of higher levels of dopamine in the synapse, which in turn is a result of accelerated firing of the presynaptic neuron.

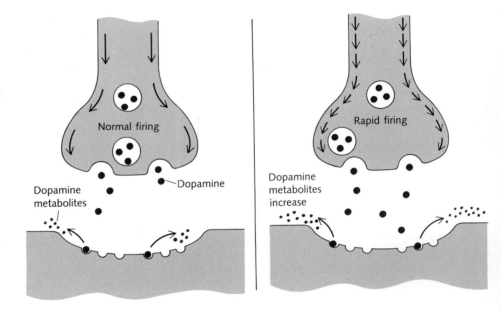

These results were puzzling. One would think that an increase in the firing rate of dopamine neurons, with more dopamine released and subsequently metabolized, would be a reflection of greater overall dopaminelike activity. Why, then, should reserpine—which causes dopamine to virtually *vanish* from the brain—have the same clinical effect as chlorpromazine—which does not affect dopamine levels but raises levels of dopamine metabolites? And how could Carlsson's results be reconciled with the fact that in Parkinson's disease dopamine neurons degenerate so that there is a corresponding dopamine *deficiency*. In attempting to resolve these seeming contradictions, Carlsson came up with the following hypothesis.

He suggested that neuroleptics block receptors for dopamine. In other words, he suggested that neuroleptics are antagonists for the neurotransmitter effects of dopamine. Accordingly, their primary action is to reduce the overall amount of dopaminelike activity in the brain. Carlsson went on to reason that the neurons with the dopamine receptors are in some sort of feedback communication with the dopamine-releasing neurons. The blockade of dopamine receptors is communicated back to the dopamine neurons with a message something like, "We are not receiving enough dopamine. Please turn on the dopamine machine!" Responding to this message, the dopamine neurons fire more rapidly and release more dopamine, and Arvid Carlsson thence detects increased levels of dopamine metabolites.

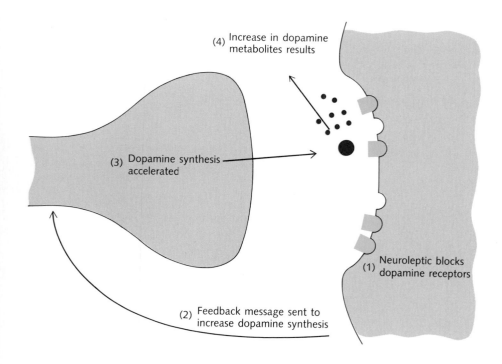

(4) Increase in dopamine metabolites results

(3) Dopamine synthesis accelerated

(1) Neuroleptic blocks dopamine receptors

(2) Feedback message sent to increase dopamine synthesis

The binding of neuroleptic drugs to dopamine receptors initiates a feedback mechanism that accelerates the firing of the presynaptic dopamine neuron.

Studying Dopamine Receptors

Carlsson's basic hypothesis was fairly straightforward: he was suggesting that neuroleptics exert their clinical actions by blocking dopamine receptors. Unfortunately, in 1962 he had no way of detecting dopamine receptors biochemically. Indeed, techniques were not then available for monitoring any neurotransmitter receptors at a molecular level.

In the years immediately following Carlsson's initial experiments, numerous scientists confirmed that neuroleptics increase the metabolism of dopamine in proportion to their clinical potencies. Researchers were even able to measure the electrical firing rate of the dopamine neurons and show that firing accelerates in animals treated with neuroleptics. But the fact remained that very little could be done to examine dopamine receptors directly. A technique that could count dopamine receptors biochemically would enable researchers to test the hypothesis that neuroleptics were indeed blocking dopamine receptors, that is, antagonizing the synaptic actions of dopamine by competing with dopamine to bind at dopamine receptors.

One of the first biochemical methods to detect the existence of dopamine receptors was developed in 1972. Paul Greengard at Yale University showed

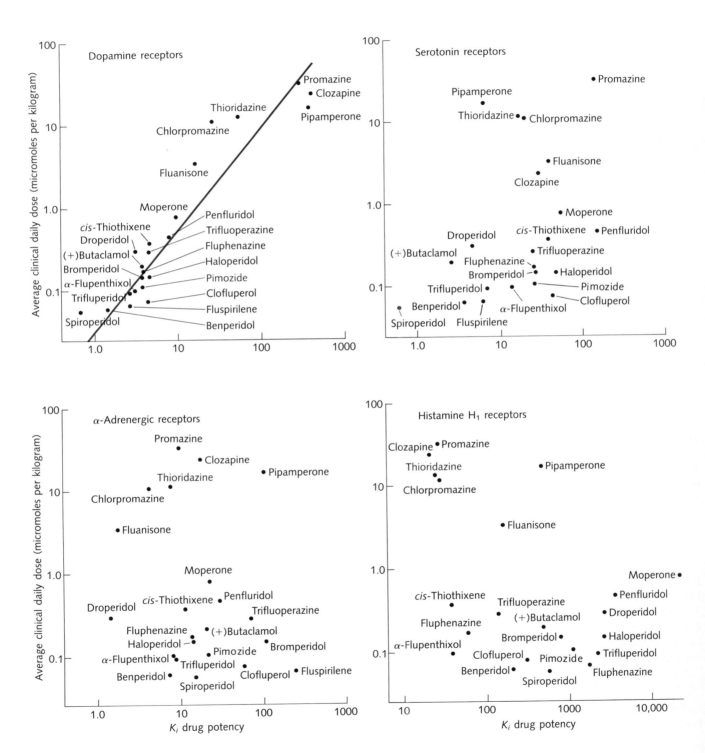

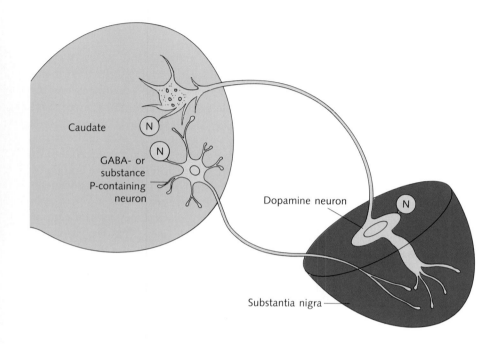

Sites at which dopamine receptors might be blocked by neuroleptic drugs (N). Catecholamine neurons are thought to have receptors distributed over all parts of their membranes.

that dopamine increases levels of cyclic AMP in the corpus striatum. Cyclic AMP, as we have seen, is a second-messenger chemical, which is to say it communicates information from a neurotransmitter receptor, in this case the dopamine receptor, to the interior of the postsynaptic nerve cell, thereby altering the rate of neuronal firing. Greengard found that when he mixed homogenates of the corpus striatum with very low concentrations of dopamine, he stimulated the formation of cyclic AMP. No other neurotransmitter he tested elicited such an effect. Greengard concluded that he was indeed monitoring an effect on neuronal metabolism that was selectively associated with dopamine actions at dopamine receptors.

Greengard also found that chlorpromazine and some of its chemical cousins blocked the ability of dopamine to stimulate cyclic AMP formation. However, there were exceptions. Haloperidol, which in clinical and animal behavioral studies had been identified as a potent neuroleptic, proved to be extremely weak in blocking dopamine effects on the level of cyclic AMP. Since haloperidol was one of the best characterized and most potent of all neuroleptics, many scientists concluded that Arvid Carlsson was wrong: neuroleptics do not act by blocking dopamine receptors. For several more years, inquiry into the relationship between dopamine and the neuroleptics remained at an impasse. Many lines of evidence favored Carlsson's theory, but his model seemed to fail the crucial test. Finally, in 1975, it became possible to identify dopamine receptors

Facing page A graph that demonstrates the correlation between the clinical potencies of neuroleptics and the drugs' blockade of dopamine receptors is compared with graphs that describe a lack of correlation between clinical potency and blockade of serotonin, alpha adrenergic, and histamine receptors.

in a direct fashion utilizing techniques that had successfully established the presence of opiate receptors.

As we saw in Chapter 2, opiate receptors were first identified in 1973, by techniques that monitored the binding of radioactive opiates to brain membranes and identified the initial opiate recognition site, the key zone where the receptor grabs hold of the drug or neurotransmitter. Biochemical alterations such as changes in cyclic AMP occur secondary to this initial receptor-binding interaction. The procedures used to identify opiate receptors provided a simple general strategy for identifying a wide range of neurotransmitter receptors. By 1975, Ian Creese and David Burt in my laboratory at Johns Hopkins and Philip Seeman at the University of Toronto had devised similar binding experiments that permitted the direct identification of dopamine receptors.

The dopamine receptors were measured in two ways. One technique monitored the binding of radioactive dopamine to membranes from dopamine-rich areas of the brain, such as the corpus striatum. When dopamine receptors were analyzed in this way, the relative abilities of various drugs to block the binding of radioactive dopamine to brain membranes were closely similar to what Greengard had observed. Chlorpromazine and several similar agents were potent dopamine blockers, and these potencies correlated well with the drugs' pharmacological activities. Thus, drugs that were more potent as antischizophrenic agents were generally more potent in blocking dopamine receptors. On the other hand, haloperidol was extremely weak.

The other technique elicited quite different results. The alternative experiments monitored the binding of radioactive haloperidol to dopamine receptors in brain membranes. We knew that the haloperidol was binding to dopamine receptors because, of all the neurotransmitters examined, only dopamine was able to compete at the binding sites. Yet, these binding sites were not the same dopamine receptors that had been labeled with radioactive dopamine. The dopamine receptors to which haloperidol bound had an extremely high affinity for haloperidol as well as an excellent affinity for chlorpromazine and other related agents. Indeed, when we evaluated the interactions of these receptors with an extensive series of neuroleptic drugs, we saw an almost perfect correlation between the affinities of neuroleptics for blocking the haloperidol-labeled dopamine receptors and the drugs' effectiveness in relieving schizophrenic symptoms. This was a most specific type of relationship. In contrast, these experiments showed us that the neuroleptics' potencies as antihistamines had no relationship to their potencies in relieving schizophrenic symptoms. Similarly, although many neuroleptics are effective in blocking norepinephrine and serotonin receptors, there was again no correlation between their effects at these sites and their antischizophrenic actions.

What could be going on? How could drug potencies at dopamine receptors vary depending on whether labeled dopamine or haloperidol was used to identify those receptors? At first we were confused by our findings, but subsequent research with a variety of neurotransmitter receptors provided a simple an-

---

Comparison of dopamine-receptor subtypes

	D_1	D_2
Prototype receptor location	Parathyroid gland	Anterior and intermediate pituitary glands
Effect on cyclic AMP levels	Increases	Decreases
Agonists:		
Dopamine	Full agonist (weak)	Full agonist (potent)
Apomorphine	Partial agonist (weak)	Full agonist (potent)
Antagonists:		
Phenothiazines	Potent	Potent
Thioxanthenes	Potent	Potent
Butyrophenones	Weak	Potent
Substituted ben- zamides	Inactive	Weak
Dopaminergic ergots	Antagonists or partial agonists (weak)	Full agonists (potent)

---

swer. Most neurotransmitters will bind to more than one type of receptor. Thus, radioactive dopamine was labeling one kind of dopamine receptor, now referred to as the D_1 receptor, while radioactive haloperidol was labeling the other type, or D_2 dopamine receptor (see the table above). In monitoring the increase in cyclic AMP, Greengard was observing a biochemical event induced by the interaction of dopamine with D_1 receptors. When interpreted in this light, his experiments showed that the antischizophrenic and Parkinson-inducing actions of neuroleptics have nothing to do with the blockade of dopamine D_1 receptors. In contrast, the extremely close correlation between a drug's pharmacological effects and its ability to block dopamine D_2 receptors indicates that Arvid Carlsson's original theory was correct. Neuroleptics do act by blocking dopamine receptors, but it is one specific subtype of dopamine receptor, the D_2 type, that is responsible.

This correlation between the clinical effects of neuroleptics and their blockade of dopamine D_2 receptors is one of the more impressive examples of pharmacological analysis. It establishes the mechanism of action for neuroleptic drugs as rigorously and as firmly as that of almost any other drug in clinical medicine.

Different Dopamine Pathways

Let us return to the initial conjecture of Delay and Deniker, namely, that neuroleptics exert a single fundamental biochemical effect that causes Parkinsonian side effects in one brain area and antischizophrenic actions in another. Since it is now established that the drugs act by blocking dopamine receptors, the next step in clarifying how neuroleptics work is to determine which parts of the brain are responsible for each type of clinical action.

Among the great advances of the past twenty years of brain research are the techniques that have enabled researchers to visualize neurotransmitters within neurons at a microscopic level. The brain contains at least fifty and perhaps as many as two hundred different neurotransmitters. Each of these is confined to specific neuronal pathways. By mapping the neuronal pathways that contain a particular neurotransmitter, scientists can make reasonable inferences about the function of that transmitter. Thus, as we saw in Chapter 2, the discovery that the opiatelike peptide neurotransmitters, the enkephalins, occupy areas of the brain that regulate pain perception and euphoria readily explained how opiates such as morphine and heroin exert their effects.

When chemical staining techniques were used to reveal dopamine-containing neuronal pathways, many questions about the role of this transmitter could be answered. The major dopamine pathway of the brain has its cell bodies in a small nucleus in the brainstem called the substantia nigra (see the figure opposite). This area is heavily pigmented with melanin and looks dark brown or black in unstained brain sections; hence its name, which in Greek means "the black substance." Its dopamine-containing nerve cells give rise to long, ascending axons that terminate with greatest densities in the corpus striatum, the part of the brain whose function is to produce a smooth coordination in the movement of arms and legs. It is this "nigrostriatal" pathway that is seen to degenerate in Parkinson's disease, disrupting motor activity and causing the characteristic rigidity, decreased movement, and tremor. Drugs cause the same symptoms in slightly different ways: reserpine, by depleting dopamine in the corpus striatum, and chlorpromazine, by blocking the dopamine receptors in that region.

A second prominent dopamine pathway has cell bodies in an area of the brainstem close to the substantia nigra and usually referred to as the ventral tegmental area, or tegmentum. Dopamine cells in this area send axons that ascend to various parts of the limbic system, a group of brain structures whose primary responsibility is the regulation of emotional behavior. These "emotional" targets of dopamine neuronal projections include the olfactory tubercle, the nucleus accumbens, and the central nucleus of the amygdala.

By its name, one can readily surmise that the olfactory tubercle has something to to with smelling behavior. Through the course of evolution, olfaction became connected with the emotions because of the importance of smell in emotionally linked behavior such as sex and identification of friends and ene-

Facing page Dopamine pathways in the human brain.

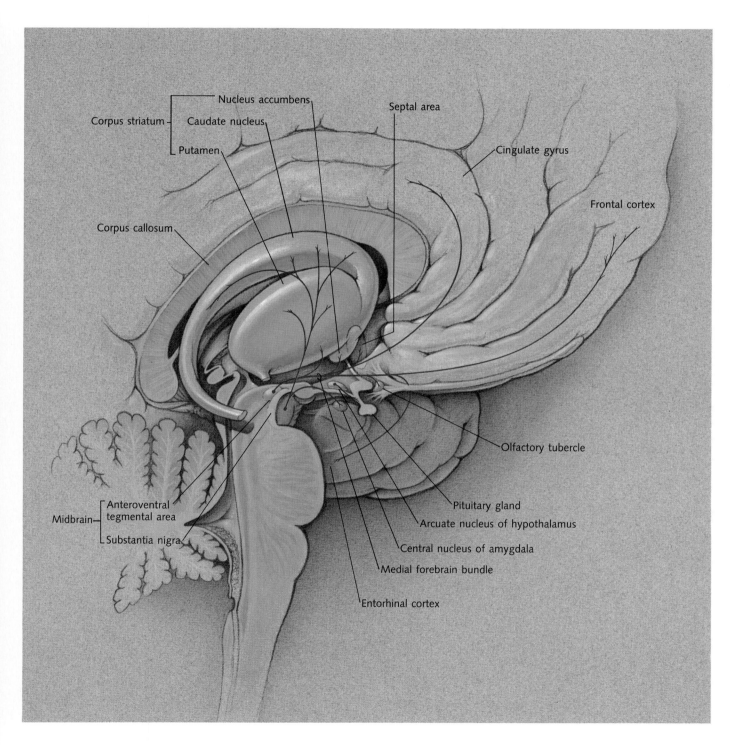

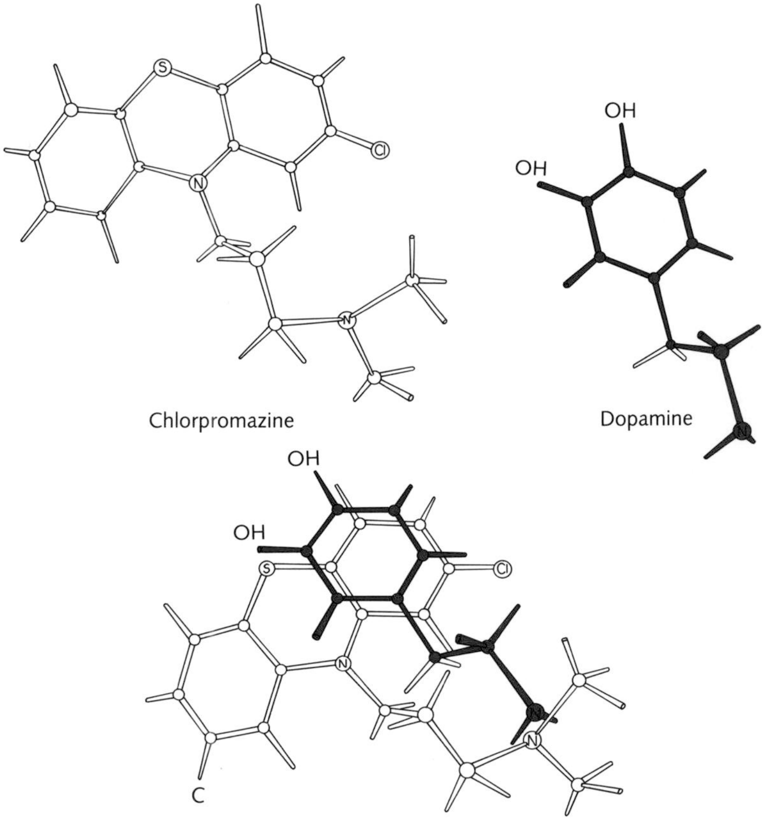

Comparison of chlorpromazine and dopamine molecular structures.

Chlorpromazine

Dopamine

C

mies. One part of the cerebral cortex, the cingulate cortex, also receives dopamine input. Interestingly, this is the "oldest" part of the cerebral cortex, judged in terms of evolutionary history, and is closely associated with the limbic system, which evolved long before the cerebral cortex. These prominent projections of dopamine neurons to limbic structures suggest that blockade of dopamine receptors in these areas accounts for the antischizophrenic actions of the drugs. That hypothesis in turn suggests that the limbic system is in some way responsible for the kinds of thought processes that go awry in schizophrenia.

There are other dopamine pathways in the brain, none of which are likely sites of antischizophrenic drug actions. One of these has its cell bodies in the hypothalamus and its axons projecting toward the pituitary gland. The hypothalamus regulates the release from the pituitary gland of hormones that influence other glands throughout the body, among them the thyroid gland, the

---

Steps in the Discovery of Neuroleptic Effects of Dopamine

1963   *Neuroleptics are seen to increase levels of dopamine metabolites*
        (Carlsson).

1972   *Dopamine is seen to stimulate cyclic AMP formation. Some neuroleptics*
        block this effect but others do not (Greengard).

1975   *Dopamine receptors are identified in binding studies. ^{3}H-Dopamine and*
        ^{3}H-haloperidol appear to label distinct sites (Burt, Creese, and
        Snyder; Seeman).

1976   *Potencies of neuroleptics in blocking D_2 dopamine receptors, labeled by*
        ^{3}H-haloperidol, correlate with therapeutic effects (Creese, Burt,
        and Snyder; Seeman).

---

adrenal gland, and the gonads. One pituitary hormone, prolactin, stimulates lactation—the secretion of milk from the breast—and inhibits hormone secretion from the ovary and testes. The firing of dopamine neurons in the hypothalamus-pituitary pathway prevents prolactin release, but in the presence of neuroleptics dopamine receptors are blocked, and the outpouring of prolactin into the bloodstream is enhanced. Not surprisingly, patients treated with neuroleptics have very high levels of prolactin in the blood and suffer from its effects. Women receiving neuroleptics are likely to begin releasing milk from their breasts and to cease menstruating. Males often show decreased sexual interest, and some are impotent.

Problems and Prospects

The discovery of neuroleptic drugs and dopamine receptors, and the analysis of their interactions in specific dopamine neuronal pathways, is one of the most remarkable tales of modern drug research. Nevertheless, the fact remains that neuroleptics are not entirely satisfactory drugs, despite their great clinical success. The drugs relieve schizophrenic symptoms, but they do not cure the disease. Patients who receive neuroleptics rarely regain "normal" mental health and must continue to take the drugs or their schizophrenic symptoms will return. Moreover, although the positive symptoms of schizophrenia—the flagrant delusions and florid hallucinations—respond dramatically to neuroleptics, the typical negative symptoms—extreme shyness and social withdrawal—do not respond very well. The distinction is so marked that some psychiatrists have suggested that different brain abnormalities are responsible for the negative and positive schizophrenic symptoms, but as yet there is no concrete evidence on this point.

If patients must receive a drug for long periods of time, then side effects become sources of great concern. Aside from the hormonal and Parkinsonian effects discussed above, schizophrenics who receive neuroleptics for many years also begin to manifest symptoms of excess dopaminelike activity. After prolonged blockade by neuroleptics, dopamine receptors seem to fight back, at least in the corpus striatum, where an actual increase in the number of dopamine receptors can be detected in animals treated chronically with neuroleptics. Whereas the dopamine deficiency of Parkinson's disease causes rigidity and diminished movement, patients who develop this superfluity and hypersensitivity of corpus striatum dopamine receptors suffer from greatly increased movements of the tongue, mouth, arms, and legs. Of particular concern is the fact that this condition, called tardive dyskinesia, does not always go away after the offending neuroleptic drug has been removed.

If dopamine-receptor sensitivity is greater in patients with tardive dyskinesia, one might wonder whether they would also suffer a corresponding increase in schizophrenic symptoms. Interestingly, though researchers have looked carefully for any possible exacerbation of schizophrenic symptoms in patients who begin to develop tardive dyskinesia, none has ever been found.

The major dilemma posed by tardive dyskinesia is the problem of developing a drug strategy for treating it while continuing to treat the schizophrenia. Increasing the dose of neuroleptics would block the augmented number of dopamine receptors, but it would also stimulate the further proliferation of dopamine receptors, which would subsequently result in yet more serious tardive dyskinesia.

At present, the greatest hope lies in the development of safer drugs. The simplest approach would be to seek agents that block dopamine receptors in the limbic parts of the brain without affecting the corpus striatum or the pituitary gland. Every year modern research techniques are dissecting receptors into more and more subtypes, and we have seen in the case of haloperidol that drugs can have a strong affinity for one subtype of a neurotransmitter receptor, and not for another. Thus far, we cannot differentiate between the dopamine D_2 receptors of the corpus striatum, the limbic system, and the pituitary gland, but the possibility of doing so is not at all that remote. The ability to study neurotransmitter receptors has enabled pharmacologists to sculpt drugs to fit particular receptors, greatly expanding the horizons of possible drug therapy in psychiatry. Hopefully, future developments will be dictated more by science than by luck.

In summary, the neuroleptics, like the opiates, are used both as therapeutic agents and as tools to help us understand brain function. They have not provided a definitive answer as to the molecular cause of schizophrenia, but the fact that they exert their therapeutic actions by blocking dopamine receptors suggests that dopamine neurons in the brain regulate mental processes relevant to the abnormalities in schizophrenic thinking. In accord with this hypothesis—and as a means of testing it—researchers all over the world are trying to analyze the behavioral functions of various dopamine neuronal pathways in the brain. While it is possible that clarifying the function of dopamine neurons will not tell us what is wrong in schizophrenic brains (perhaps the defect lies elsewhere, with dopamine merely modulating the abnormal site), nonetheless, research on neuroleptics and dopamine has provided us with powerful probes to attack the key questions relating to the cause of the dreaded disease. In the next chapter, we will see how, prompted by the remarkable progress that has been achieved with antischizophrenics, scientists developed quite a different form of drug therapy to treat another serious form of mental illness.

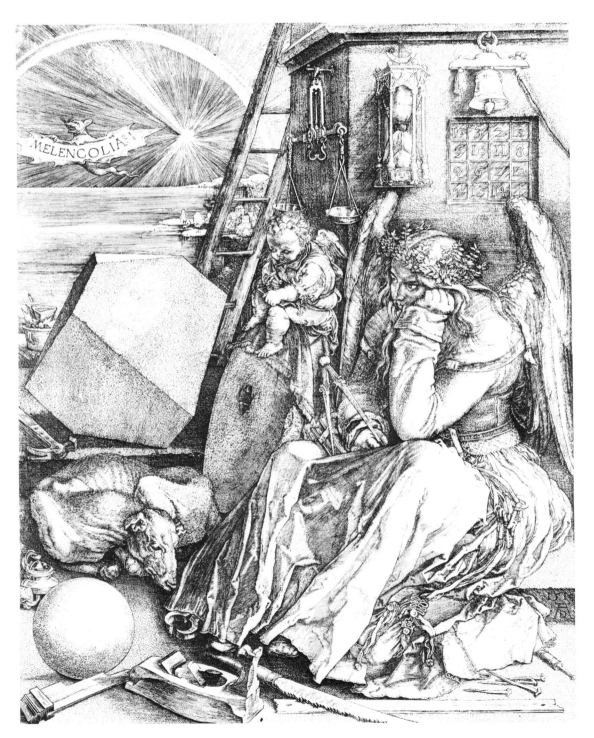

MELENCOLIA§I

4 | Mood Modifiers

The Greek biographer Plutarch has been called a skillful writer who did not hesitate to improve on history when the facts were lacking in drama. Nevertheless, he was an astute observer of reality, and his description of a man in the depths of depression is entirely true to life: "He sits out of doors, wrapped in sack cloth or in filthy rags. Ever anon he rolls himself naked in the dirt confessing about this or that sin. He has eaten or drunk something wrong. He has gone some way or other which the Divine Being did not approve of." Plutarch conveys the intense psychic pain of depression with more clarity and poignance than one would find in a typically impassive clinical report; at the same time, as we will see, he touches on a number of the diagnostic symptoms.

All of us know the feeling of being depressed. When we suffer the loss of a close friend or relative through death or divorce, or simply through removal to a distance, all of us are likely to feel dejected. When something damages our self-esteem, when we lose a job or fail a course in school, it is common to question our self-worth, to feel "blue," and to lose interest in friends and everyday activities. What, then, do psychiatrists mean when they designate a patient as suffering from the "disease" of depression? Is there a specific biological abnormality, as concrete as a bacterial infection, or is depression part of a continuum that ranges from the everyday sadness we all experience to the extremes of abject hopelessness that lead to suicide?

As yet, there are no definite answers. However, evidence from genetic studies, which we will review below, indicates that certain forms of depression represent genuine disease entities quite distinct from the sadness that everyone experiences now and then. The depth of misery of the seriously depressed patient is much more intense than any "normal" unhappiness. I find it difficult to describe the extraordinary psychic pain that I have sensed in many of my patients. One way of capturing this mental state is to read the words of those victims who had the talent to communicate their anguish in writing. Some examples are presented on the following page.

Facing page Melencolia I, by Albrecht Dürer.

Personal Accounts of Depression

"My first impression was that something had sneaked up on me. I had no idea I was depressed, that is, mentally. I knew I felt bad, I knew I felt low. I knew I had no faith in the work I was doing or the people I was working with, but I didn't imagine I was sick. It was a great burden to get up in the morning and I couldn't wait to go to bed at night, even though I started not sleeping well . . . . I thought I was well but feeling low because of a hidden personal discouragement of some sort—something I couldn't quite put my finger on . . . . I just forced myself to live through a dreary, hopeless existence that lasted for months on end before it switched out of the dark-blue mood and into a brighter color. But even then I didn't know I had been ill." —Joshua Logan, theatrical producer and director

"The truth lay in this—that life had no meaning for me. Every day of life, every step in it, brought me nearer the edge of a precipice, whence I saw clearly the final ruin before me. To stop, to go back, were alike impossible; nor could I shut my eyes so as not to see the suffering that alone awaited me, the death of all in me, even to annihilation. Thus I, a healthy and happy man, was brought to feel that I could live no longer, that an irresistible force was dragging me down into the grave." —Leo Tolstoy, novelist and philosopher

"After all this, I have to admit that I am a failed suicide . . . . I built up to the act carefully and for a long time, with a kind of blank pertinacity . . . . Each sporadic burst of work, each minor success and disappointment, each moment of calm and relaxation, seemed merely a temporary halt on my steady descent through layer after layer of depression, like an elevator stopping for a moment on the way down to the basement . . . .

". . . My life felt so cluttered and obstructed that I could hardly breathe. I inhabited a closed, concentrated world, airless and without exits. I doubt if any of this was noticeable socially: I was simply more tense, more nervous than usual, and I drank more. But underneath I was going a bit mad." —A. Alvarez, poet and critic

"It strikes me—what are these sudden fits of complete exhaustion? I come in here to write; can't even finish a sentence; and am pulled under; now is this some odd effort; the subconscious pulling me down into her? I've been reading Faber on Newman; compared his account of a nervous breakdown; the refusal of some part of the mechanism; is that what happens to me? Not quite. Because I'm not evading anything. I long to write The Pargiters. *No. I think the effort to live in two spheres: the novel; and life; is a strain . . . . To have to behave with circumspection and decision to strangers wrenches me into another region; hence the collapse."*
—Virginia Woolf, novelist, critic, and essayist

"Only I wasn't steering anything, not even myself. I just bumped from my hotel to work and to parties and from parties to my hotel and back to work like a numb trolleybus. I guess I should have been excited the way most of the other girls were, but I couldn't get myself to react. I felt very still and very empty, the way the eye of a tornado must feel, moving dully along in the middle of the surrounding hullabaloo."   —Sylvia Plath, novelist and poet

Like the man in Plutarch's description, most depressed individuals suffer so much emotional agony for no apparent reason that they torture their minds to discover possible explanations, sins they may have committed or powerful authorities they may have angered. His own unhappiness led the British writer John Custance to conclude, "For some inscrutable reason, perhaps because I had committed the unforgiveable sin or just because I was such an appalling sinner, the worse man who ever existed, I had been chosen to go alive through the portals of hell."

Depression is only one form a mood disorder can take. Mania is the other side of the coin. Generally speaking, manic individuals are elated, full of energy, and ever optimistic, although like depressive patients, they, too, exhibit symptoms of varying severity. In a mild state of mania, called hypomania, patients can function reasonably well at work and in family relationships; indeed, some people live most of their lives in a state of perpetual hypomania. The trouble begins when a manic enters a state of excessive excitement. Judgment begins to fail, and patients become wildly extravagant in everything they say and do. This can mean flagrant sexual promiscuity, incredibly impulsive spending sprees, and incessant talking in which sentences run end on end in what psychiatrists refer to as a "flight of ideas." Manics sleep little, sometimes not at all. They bounce out of bed, after two or three hours of sleep, full of energy and new projects, but in their excited state they lack the concentration to carry these plans to a successful conclusion.

Patterns of Depression and Mania

States of mania frequently alternate with states of depression in the same individual. This condition is called a bipolar affective disorder, indicating that the patient suffers from an instability of affect, or feeling state, that can scale the poles of depression and mania. Bipolar illness is one of the two major psychotic disorders, the other being schizophrenia, the illness we discussed in Chapter 3.

The pattern of alternation between mania and depression may vary, but the depression intervals usually last longer than the periods of mania (although the latter exhibit quite a range of duration, from two hours to two years). In the absence of treatment, it is not unusual for depressed episodes to last as long as a year or even longer. Many patients have frequent depressive spells with normal intervals in between and suffer manic attacks only rarely. Others experience mania more often than depression. A most remarkable group of patients cycle from one pole to the other in almost clocklike fashion for years on end. Cases have been reported in which manic and depressive episodes of precise numbers of days followed one another with such regularity that the patient's family could predict one or two years in advance the mental state of their afflicted relative on any given date. There are families who plan summer vacations over a year in advance, aiming for the particular two-week period when, say, the bipolar father could be expected to be mildly hypomanic, ideal for a summer outing. This clocklike rhythm strongly suggests the presence of biologically determined disease. Moreover, abundant genetic evidence argues that the overall disturbance has a strong genetic component.

Many depressed patients suffer repeated episodes of depression but never experience any mania. These patients are said to have a unipolar affective disturbance, a disease entity in its own right that differs in many ways from bipolar depression. Bipolar individuals tend to become ill at an earlier age than unipolar patients. When bipolar patients are depressed, they are usually more disabled and abject, hardly moving about and seemingly unaware of anything going on in their vicinity. On the other hand, unipolar patients are more likely to be anxious and agitated, pacing the floor and crying but continuing to react to their surroundings and to interact with those about them.

Affective disorders are remarkably common. The incidence of manic-depressive illness in the general population is approximately 2 or 3 percent, about two to three times more common than severe schizophrenia. As with schizophrenia, manic-depressive illness is not unique to any particular culture. Studies conducted in wealthy and poor societies, in northern climates and tropical ones, and in capitalist and communist nations invariably show much the same incidence.

It is a little more difficult to develop comparable incidence figures for unipolar illness since different researchers may employ somewhat different diagnostic criteria to distinguish a clinically significant depression from one that is a normal response to trauma. However, the approximate instance of unipolar depression in the general population is 5 percent and appears to be fairly constant in most societies.

Family studies indicate that genetic factors play a major role in determining the likelihood of a person's becoming manic and/or depressed. The studies also show clear-cut differences in the distribution of bipolar and unipolar illnesses. For instance, in one study, 20 percent of first-degree relatives (brothers, sisters, parents, and children) of bipolar patients had bipolar illness while less than 1 percent had unipolar illness. With unipolar patients, the opposite pattern was apparent: almost 10 percent of first-degree relatives had unipolar illness and less than half a percent had bipolar. Evidently, bipolar and unipolar depressions are separate, genetically influenced diseases that run in different families.

These family studies provide the strongest grounds for believing that certain forms of mania and depression are biological entities. Particularly convincing evidence comes from investigations of twins. As we saw when we discussed genetic patterns of schizophrenia in Chapter 3, identical twins emerge from the same fertilized egg and have identical genetic endowments, whereas fraternal twins are genetically no more similar than ordinary siblings. In twin studies, the bipolar form of depression displays a stronger genetic component than does the unipolar form. If one of a pair of identical twins develops manic-depressive disease, the other twin has more than a 60-percent likelihood of becoming manic-depressive as well. The corresponding concordance rate for fraternal twins is only 10 to 20 percent, which is the same as the concordance rate for siblings who are not twins. In contrast to these statistics for bipolar depression, the concordance rate for unipolar illness is about 40 percent in identical twins and 10 to 15 percent in fraternal twins or ordinary siblings.

As in the studies of schizophrenia, one wonders why the concordance rate in identical twins is not 100 percent. Clearly, the presumed genetic abnormality merely confers a vulnerability to develop the disorder. Later, some environmental factor determines whether the genetic vulnerability will be expressed in clinical symptoms. For the affective disorders, the contributing environmental factors have not yet been pinpointed.

The twin studies resembled the other family studies of depression in that if both twins in a family were affected, they usually had the same kind of depression: either both had bipolar, that is, manic-depressive, disorder or both had unipolar disease. This again highlights the likelihood that bipolar and unipolar depressions are separate illnesses, as does the fact that twin studies show unipolar illness to have a much more limited genetic loading than does bipolar disease.

Antidepressants Discovered

Scientists and physicians have searched since the days of Hippocrates for effective ways to treat depression. Opiates were widely used for many years, but the euphoria they produce is too short-lived to be of practical use in relieving depression. Moreover, once the patient becomes addicted, his or her depression gets worse than ever. Complex alcoholic concoctions have also been employed, but these, too, brought only temporary relief and over the long term caused the depressed state to worsen. Many present-day depressives turn to alcohol for relief and in consequence develop a drinking problem that only serves to mask the depression. Clinicians may then think they are dealing with a patient whose primary problem is alcoholism, when in fact the fundamental disturbance is depression, and the alcoholism is only an external manifestation.

The need for a satisfactory means of treating depression is especially urgent because of the very real likelihood that the depressed patient will try to commit suicide. Almost every seriously depressed individual has contemplated suicide, and large numbers have successfully carried out the act. The incidence of suicidal death in diagnosed manic-depressive illness is 5 to 10 percent, higher than the suicide incidence for any other type of psychiatric illness. The incidence of suicide is only 2 percent in severe forms of schizophrenia, while for the population in general, it is a small fraction of 1 percent.

Considering the perilous situation of the severely depressed patient, his or her treating physician is often under great stress. Imagine, then, the difficulty and misery that doctors and patients faced before the advent of antidepressant drugs, when each period of crisis was likely to last up to a year or more! Not surprisingly, the discovery of the modern antidepressant drugs has been regarded as a great blessing to medicine in general and to the practice of psychiatry in particular.

As in the case of the antischizophrenic drugs, discovery of the antidepressants involved large doses of serendipity coupled with occasional flashes of brilliant scientific insight. Interestingly, it was the advent of the antischizophrenics that provided renewed impetus to the search for an antidepressant agent and that directed researchers' efforts toward an area of inquiry that finally yielded some exciting results.

The first class of antidepressant drugs to be introduced were the monoamine oxidase inhibitors. The name reflects their primary physiological activity, which is to inhibit an enzyme called monoamine oxidase; however, at the time iproniazid, the parent drug in this class, was discovered, no one knew that it affected monoamine oxidase or that such an effect would have anything to do with depression. In fact, iproniazid was originally introduced to the medical market, in the early 1950s, as a treatment for tuberculosis, and as such it was not a particular success. Luckily, circumstances conspired to bring iproniazid to the attention of psychiatrist Nathan Kline, who had pieced together important clues from various sources. One clue had to do with iproniazid experiments in rats.

By the mid-1950s, studies of the effects of drugs on the behavior of rats had become commonplace. The success of reserpine and chlorpromazine in treat-

Isoniazid

Iproniazid

ing schizophrenia had prompted researchers all over the world to study the drugs' effects in animals in order to analyze their mechanisms of action. The first task in this endeavor was to find some model of animal behavior that could be used as an analogue of certain schizophrenic behaviors. For example, when reserpine is given to rats, they become sluggish and move around very little. Scientists wondered whether this might be regarded as analogous to the effects of reserpine in reducing some of the more florid, hyperactive symptoms of schizophrenia. Of course, they had no idea what the rats were feeling or thinking and might just as well have compared the reserpine-treated rats to severely depressed patients as to schizophrenic ones. Nevertheless, tests on rats continued as scientists strove to find a solution to this dilemma.

It was already known that reserpine depletes the brain of the biogenic amines norepinephrine and serotonin. Impressed with that striking effect, scientists were interested in finding other drugs that had a marked influence on brain chemicals. Albert Zeller, a biochemist working out of Northwestern University, had discovered that the enzyme monoamine oxidase removes the amine grouping from amine neurotransmitters, including norepinephrine and serotonin, and he suggested that this might be the way the body normally inactivates those compounds after their synaptic transmission has been accomplished. He began to screen a number of chemicals to see if any would inhibit the enzyme and thus possibly increase the levels of amine neurotransmitters in the brain. Iproniazid was one of the compounds Zeller obtained from various drug companies, and he found that it rather potently inhibited the activity of monoamine oxidase.

Several scientists decided to test the effects of iproniazid on rats. First they determined the biochemical effects of the drug. This meant administering the drug to rats, killing them, and, by means of standard chemical techniques, ascertaining that iproniazid did indeed elevate levels of norepinephrine and serotonin in the rats' brains. The next step was to examine the behavior of rats treated with iproniazid alone and then with combinations of iproniazid and reserpine. Because reserpine, an antischizophrenic agent, was known to lower brain concentrations of the amines and iproniazid had been seen to raise them, researchers hoped that testing the drugs in combination would provide an indication of what iproniazid might do in schizophrenic patients. Treatment with iproniazid alone seemed to have little effect on the rats' behavior, but rats that became almost immobile when treated with reserpine alone became hyperactive, running to and fro across the cage, when treated with a combination of reserpine and iproniazid (see the graph on page 98).

The apparent excitation produced in rats by the combination of iproniazid and reserpine suggested that iproniazid might reverse the antischizophrenic effects of reserpine in humans. On the other hand, it was possible that the excited state displayed by the rats could instead reflect a "psychic energizing" action of iproniazid that might be useful in treating depression.

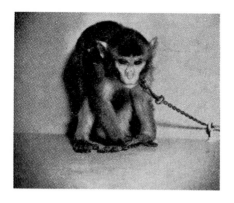

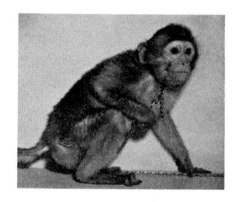

Use of reserpine as a laboratory model of depression. A normal alert monkey shows signs of depression 4 hours after receiving 10 milligrams per kilogram of reserpine (*top*). Drug researchers test possible antidepressants by examining their effects on reserpine-induced depression. In this case, the monkey resumed normal behavior (*bottom*) after it was treated with a combination of pargyline and dopa. Pargyline is an antidepressant drug that acts by inhibiting monoamine oxidase.

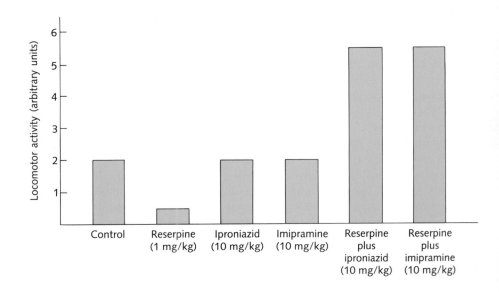

Effects of reserpine, iproniazid, and imipramine on rat locomotor activity. Note the marked increase in activity following administration of reserpine in combination with iproniazid or imipramine.

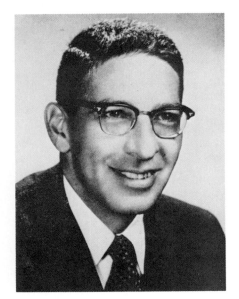

Nathan Kline (1916–1984), the psychiatrist who discovered the antidepressant action of iproniazid.

One piece of evidence favoring the latter possibility came from the clinical studies in which iproniazid was used to treat tuberculosis. Some physicians reported that their patients became euphoric. Of course, recovery from a condition as debilitating as tuberculosis would surely raise a patient's spirits, but the elation of the iproniazid-treated patients seemed out of all proportion to what doctors had come to expect from patients who had been cured of their disease.

Late in 1956, these considerations led Nathan Kline to begin treating hospitalized schizophrenics with iproniazid either alone or in combination with reserpine. He also commenced giving iproniazid to some of the depressed patients he was seeing in his private office practice. Within a month, Kline observed dramatic improvement in his depressed patients but signs of deterioration in the schizophrenic ones. His observations very quickly led to widespread use of iproniazid as an antidepressant. The fact that the drug was already being marketed in the United States as a treatment for tuberculosis greatly facilitated its extension to psychiatry. Within a year, hundreds of thousands of depressed patients were being treated with iproniazid.

How Monoamine Oxidase Inhibitors Work

The clinical success of iproniazid sparked the drug industry to develop dozens of other drugs that, like iproniazid, inhibit the action of the enzyme monoamine oxidase. All proved to be effective antidepressants, confirming the theory that inhibition of this enzyme was a key to the relief of depression. Scientists have since found partial reasons for this phenomenon. For one thing, they soon discovered why treating rats with monoamine oxidase inhibitors converts the reserpine-induced "depression" into hyperactivity.

By the early 1960s it was known that reserpine depletes the brain of norepinephrine and serotonin by causing these transmitter molecules to leak out of the synaptic vesicles in which they are stored. As soon as they leak out of the vesicles, which as you will recall are located in the nerve endings, the transmitters are exposed to monoamine oxidase contained within the same nerve endings. Under normal circumstances, monoamine oxidase acts as a "safety valve" to degrade any excess transmitter molecules that may spill out of synaptic vesicles when the neuron is in a resting state. Monoamine oxidase inhibitors prevent this inactivation. In their presence, any neurotransmitter molecules that leak out of the synaptic vesicles survive to enter the synapse intact (see the diagram below). Receptors for norepinephrine and serotonin are thus exposed to a great excess of these transmitters, a circumstance that somehow provokes behavioral excitation. Virtually every clinically effective antidepressant reverses reserpine-induced sedation, increasing brain levels of norepinephrine and serotonin in the process. Although the exact mechanism of monoamine oxidase inhibition effects on depression is not known, the ability of a drug to reverse reserpine-induced sedation has turned out to be a powerful predictor of

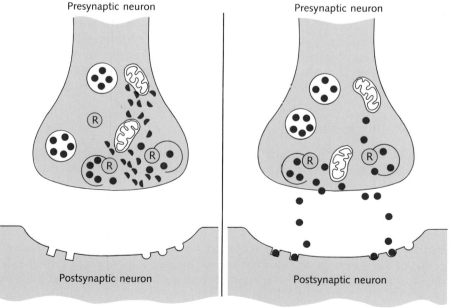

Left Reserpine (R) causes norepinephrine and serotonin to leak out of synaptic vesicles in the nerve ending. No longer protected by the storage vesicles, the neurotransmitters are degraded by monoamine oxidase. *Right* The presence of monoamine oxidase inhibitors prevents neurotransmitter degradation. Neurotransmitter molecules diffuse into the synapse and bind to receptors on the adjacent neuron.

Monoamine oxidase (MAO) is the enzyme responsible for the oxidative deamination of norepinephrine and serotonin.

Norepinephrine

Serotonin

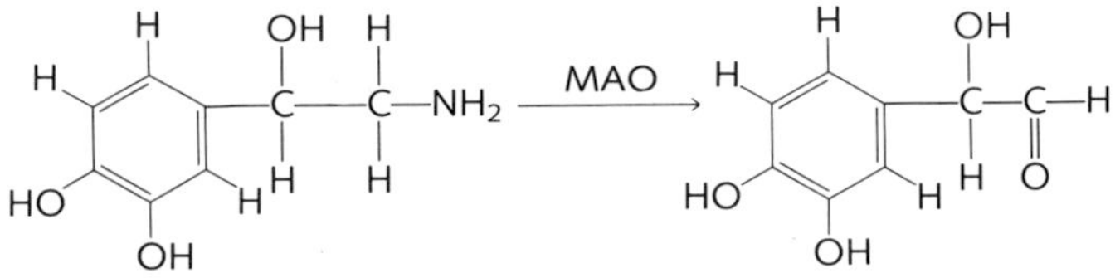

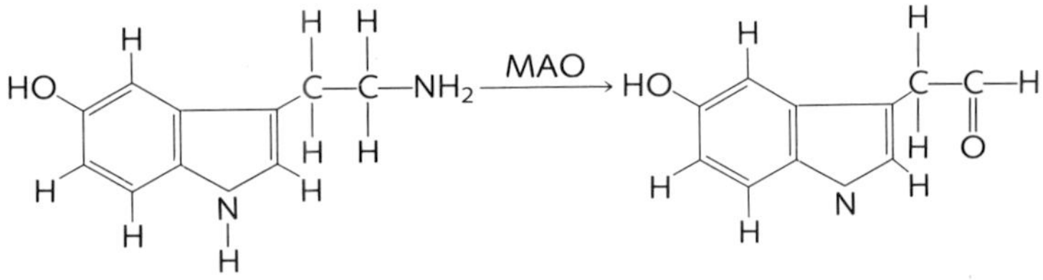

whether it will be an effective antidepressant. Drug companies have made extensive use of this model as a screening test for new antidepressants.

Even before they had managed to explain the antidepressant actions of the monoamine oxidase inhibitors, researchers knew that the end result of those actions was an elevation in the levels of norepinephrine and serotonin in the brain. Psychiatrists had already been considering what that might suggest about the brain chemistry of seriously depressed patients. Perhaps depression resulted from abnormally low levels of these amine neurotransmitters; or, if the levels were normal, perhaps the transmitters were functionally deficient in some way. This "amine hypothesis" aroused considerable interest. We will return to it later, after discussing what the discovery of a second class of antidepressants was able to contribute to our knowledge of depression.

Tricyclic Antidepressants

Monoamine oxidase inhibitors were the first widely used antidepressants, but because of various undesirable side effects, they are employed today in only a limited number of cases. The most serious side effect concerns the interaction of the monoamine oxidase inhibitors with certain foods. Tyramine, an amine present in cheese, wine, pickled foods, and other fare, is a powerful elevator of blood pressure. Because this amine is normally metabolized by monoamine oxidase in the liver, most people can eat tyramine-containing foods without concern, but when patients on monoamine oxidase inhibitors eat those foods, they run a risk of developing abrupt, pronounced increases in blood pressure

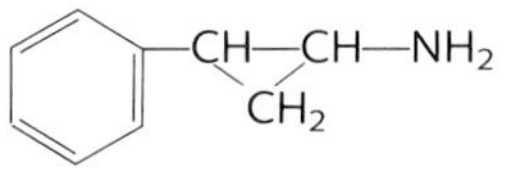

CH—CH—NH₂ ... CH₂

Tranylcypromine

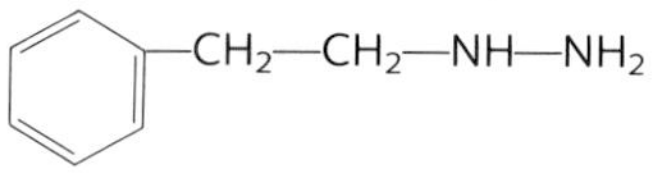

CH₂—CH₂—NH—NH₂

Phenelzine

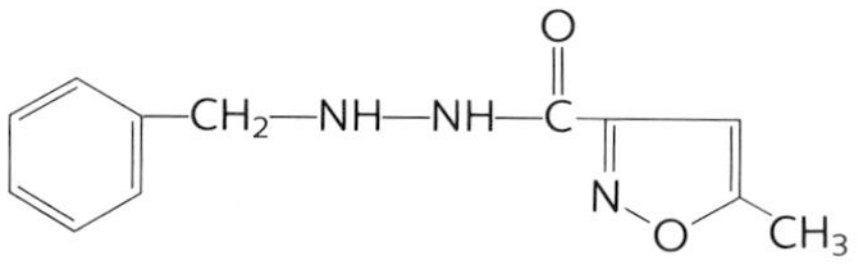

CH₂—NH—NH—C

Isocarboxazid

CH₃

Chemical structures of MAO inhibitor antidepressants.

that can lead to lethal hemorrhages in the brain. Fortunately, another group of antidepressant drugs has been developed to take the place of the monoamine oxidase inhibitors. These drugs are called tricyclics, because all have chemical structures resembling a three-ring chain. Some representative tricyclic drugs are depicted on page 102.

The clinical actions of monoamine oxidase inhibitors and tricyclic antidepressants are quite similar. In normal, nondepressed people, the drugs do very little other than cause a mild degree of sedation. Occasionally, some monoamine oxidase inhibitors produce a stimulated state in normal subjects, similar to the state induced by amphetamines, but this is not common. When depressed patients are treated with either class of antidepressants, however, clinical improvement is marked, but there is usually a lag period of about two weeks before any changes are observed. Researchers have tried hard to understand the reasons for this lag period but with no major success. In any case, after the lag period, all the major symptoms of depression begin gradually to disappear. In many instances, nurses will notice that a patient is more active physically and more interactive socially even though the patient still denies "feeling" better. The similarity in all these details between the behavioral effects of the two types of antidepressants suggests that the underlying mechanisms of action must be similar.

The history of the tricyclic antidepressants is far less convoluted than that of the monoamine oxidase inhibitors. Imipramine, the parent tricyclic drug, was synthesized as a me-too follow-up to chlorpromazine, whose great success as an antischizophrenic agent had sparked efforts in pharmaceutical companies to develop successors that might be more effective or at least have fewer side effects. Chlorpromazine (illustrated on page 102) has a three-ring structure and a side chain with a nitrogen atom as its end. The side chain ending with nitrogen appeared to be critical to the drug's antischizophrenic activity, so chemists originally left that part of the molecule intact. Instead, they tested the

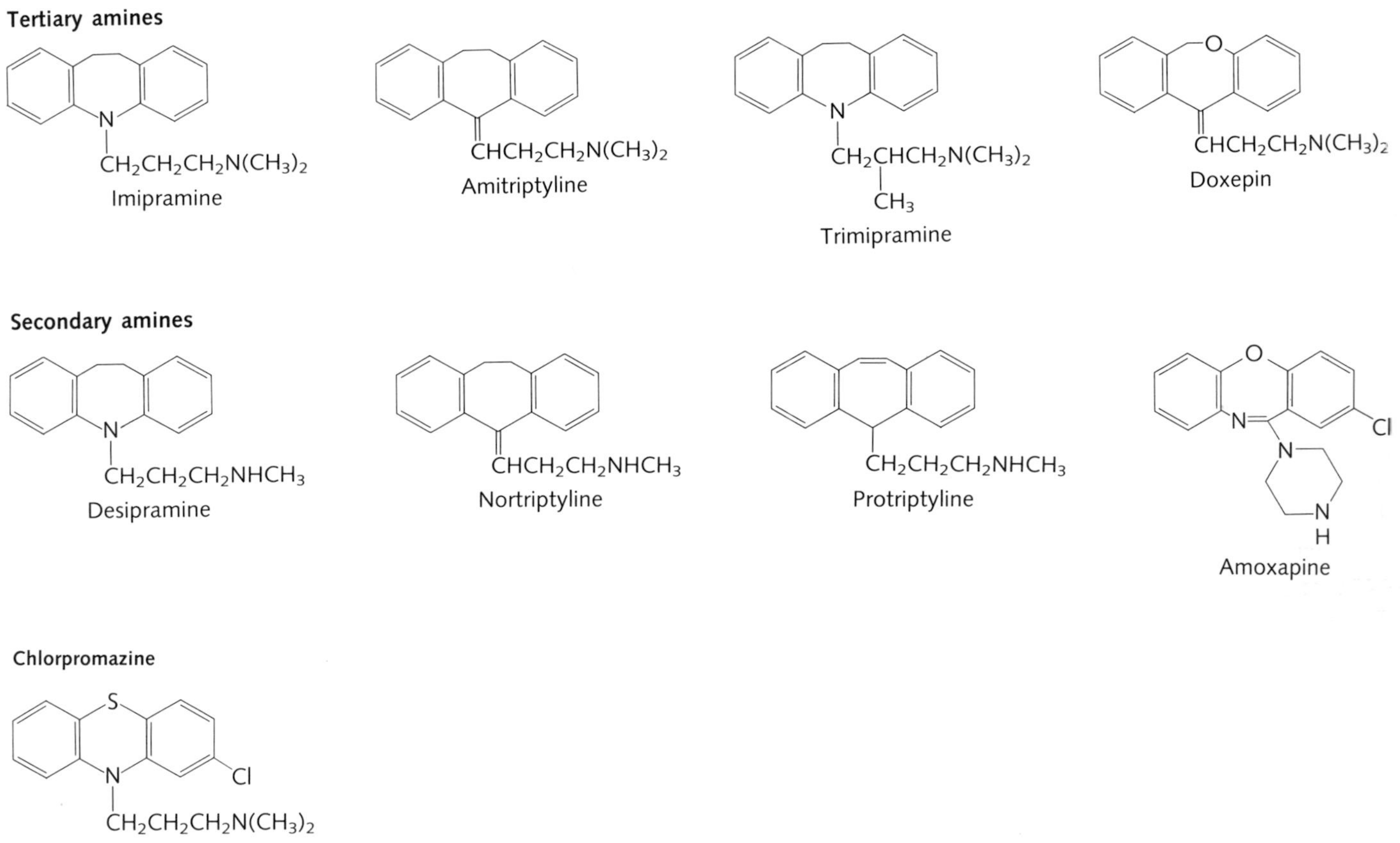

Tertiary amines

Imipramine

Amitriptyline

Trimipramine

Doxepin

Secondary amines

Desipramine

Nortriptyline

Protriptyline

Amoxapine

Chlorpromazine

Chemical structures of tricyclic antidepressants (first two rows) and chlorpromazine. Tertiary amines are so called because they have three carbons attached to the nitrogen atom in the side chain; secondary amines have two.

effects of making various modifications in the ring system. Chlorpromazine is somewhat unstable because the sulfur atom in its middle ring oxidizes readily. Accordingly, variants were synthesized in which sulfur was replaced by other atoms, such as carbon. Imipramine was one of these variants.

In 1955, the Geigy Drug Company in Basel, Switzerland, gave samples of imipramine to a Swiss psychiatrist named Roland Kuhn. This was before monoamine oxidase inhibitors were known to be antidepressants. Kuhn administered the drug to almost three hundred schizophrenics but was unable to detect any improvement. As an antischizophrenic, imipramine was clearly no match for the highly effective chlorpromazine, so it is remarkable that Kuhn persisted in testing it through so many patients. His desire to do a thorough job was of such heroic proportions, that instead of giving up he next tested the drug in other diagnostic categories, including patients with severe depression. Kuhn's tenaciousness was rewarded. In his own words, "After treating our first three cases, it was already clear to us that the substance G22355, later known as imipramine, had an antidepressive action." Studies of larger numbers of patients by Kuhn and other psychiatrists confirmed these initial findings. The Geigy Company moved quickly: by the spring of 1958, imipramine was on the market, roughly a year after the introduction of iproniazid.

Tests showed that imipramine and related drugs were extremely weak if not completely inactive as inhibitors of the enzyme monoamine oxidase. Nevertheless, the behavioral effects of imipramine and the other tricyclic antidepressants were so similar to those of the monoamine oxidase inhibitors that researchers thought the tricyclics might be elevating levels of norepinephrine or serotonin in some other way. Therefore, when tests in rats showed that imipramine did *not* increase brain levels of any neurotransmitters, the investigation arrived at an impasse. Many scientists were ready to discard the theory that biogenic amines were responsible for antidepressant drug effects, but others, equally perplexed, persisted in the belief that the amine hypothesis would prove to be correct and that imipramine must therefore have something to do with the amine neurotransmitters.

Another Form of Neurotransmitter Inactivation

At just about this time, advances in understanding synaptic transmission provided some welcome clues to the molecular basis of tricyclic antidepressant effects. Research had brought to light another mechanism for the inactivation of neurotransmitters after they have been released from recognition sites.

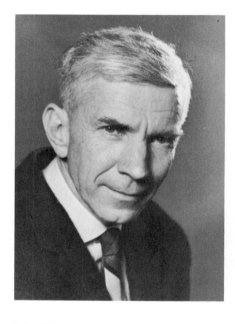

Roland Kuhn (1912–   ), the Swiss psychiatrist who discovered the antidepressant effects of imipramine.

As discussed in Chapter 1, acetylcholine was the first substance to be identified as a neurotransmitter, and scientists had eventually learned that the synaptic actions of acetylcholine are terminated by the enzyme acetylcholinesterase. This enzyme is located close to the acetylcholine receptors, where it can pounce upon acetylcholine molecules immediately after they have bound to receptors and changed the firing rate of the cell. Acetylcholinesterase cuts the acetylcholine molecule almost literally in half, destroying the neurotransmitter's ability to activate receptors. Drugs that inhibit acetylcholinesterase invariably potentiate the synaptic effects of acetylcholine.

Based on the precedent set by acetylcholine, scientists assumed that all neurotransmitters are inactivated by enzymes that degrade them. When monoamine oxidase was discovered, it was therefore only logical to expect it to perform an analogous function, that of inactivating amines such as norepinephrine, serotonin, and dopamine after they have crossed the synapse and bound at receptor sites. However, scientists soon encountered problems with this model. For one thing, when an amine neurotransmitter was applied directly to a synapse, the effects upon receptor sites were not potentiated in the presence of monoamine oxidase inhibitors. Moreover, later experiments revealed that monoamine oxidase itself is not located adjacent to neuronal receptors the way acetylcholinesterase is known to be. Instead, the bulk of monoamine oxidase in the nervous system is located in the walls of mitochondria, a species of subcellular particle confined *within* the neurons. Mitochondria are organelles found in the cytoplasm of most types of cells, including nerve cells; they play an important role in generating the energy needed by the cell (see the schematic drawing of the nerve ending on page 8). When reserpine treatment causes amine molecules to leak out of their synaptic vesicles, the molecules are degraded by monoamine oxidase situated in the walls of nearby mitochondria. Since these discoveries showed that monoamine oxidase was not responsible for the synaptic inactivation of amine neurotransmitters, scientists began to search, on the one hand, for another enzyme that might destroy the transmitters and, on the other, for an alternative inactivating mechanism that did not involve enzymes.

Julius Axelrod, who was to win the Nobel Prize in medicine in 1970, made important advances toward resolving this predicament. In the late 1950s Axelrod was working in a small laboratory at the National Institutes of Health in Bethesda, Maryland. There he began to examine the role of norepinephrine as a neurotransmitter in the sympathetic nervous system, a part of the nervous

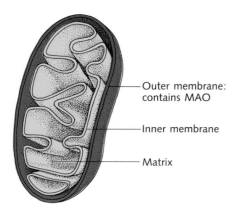

A nerve cell mitochondrion. Mitochondria are the subcellular organelles whose principal function is to break down large energy-yielding nutrient molecules into smaller packages for use in the cell.

Outer membrane: contains MAO

Inner membrane

Matrix

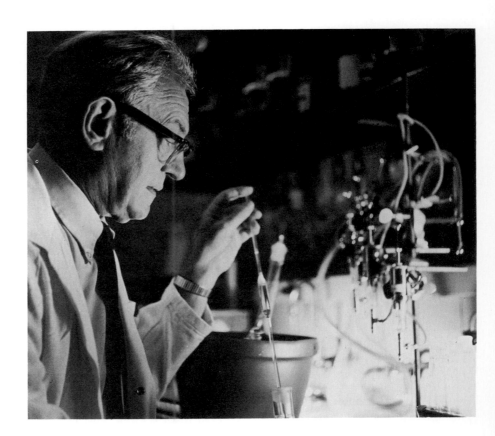

Julius Axelrod (1912–   ) discovered the mechanism by which most neurotransmitters in the brain normally are inactivated.

system that acts upon many glands and involuntary muscles, helping to regulate the body's internal environment. When sympathetic nerves are activated, which occurs mostly during periods of stress and danger, the release of their neurotransmitter, norepinephrine, causes the heart rate to speed up, the sweat glands to be stimulated, and additional amounts of blood to flow toward the muscles. These are all adjustments that prepare an organism to deal with a dangerous situation.

Axelrod's plan was to administer radioactively labeled norepinephrine to animals and monitor its disposition in their bodies by counting the radioactivity in different tissues. (He had been provided with the first batches of synthetic tritium-labeled norepinephrine ever produced; tritium is another name for radioactive hydrogen). Axelrod discovered that the tritium-labeled norepinephrine was rapidly accumulated in tissues known to have large numbers of sympathetic nerve endings. The heart is one example; the spleen is another. When he cut the sympathetic nerve, so that the nerve endings degenerated, the norepinephrine no longer accumulated in those tissues, an indication that the sympathetic nerve endings had been absorbing the injected tritium-labeled norepinephrine (see the diagram below). After the sympathetic nerves had been cut, Axelrod also observed that the physiological effects that generally follow an injection of norepinephrine—the rise in blood pressure, sudden perspiration, and so forth—were greatly enhanced. He concluded that a norepinephrine-uptake mechanism in sympathetic nerve cell endings normally inactivates the norepinephrine released at their synapses.

Axelrod subsequently showed that the nerve endings of norepinephrine-containing neurons in the brain inactivate norepinephrine by the same pump-like mechanism as the nerve endings of norepinephrine neurons in the sympa-

When Axelrod injected tritium-labeled norepinephrine into rats, the radioactive substance accumulated in organs known to have large numbers of sympathetic nerve endings. When the sympathetic nerve branches were cut, norepinephrine no longer collected in those tissues.

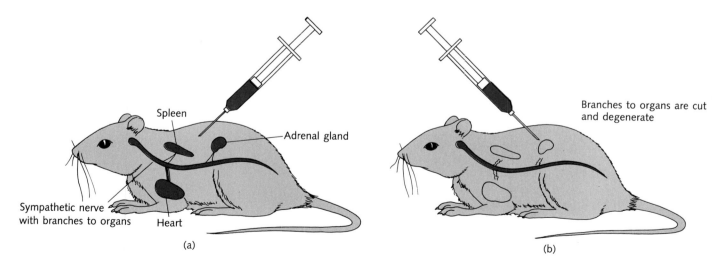

Spleen — Adrenal gland — Sympathetic nerve with branches to organs — Heart (a) — Branches to organs are cut and degenerate (b)

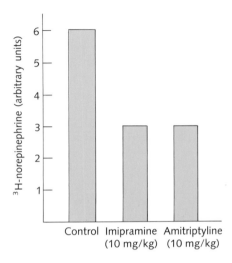

Axelrod found that tricyclic antidepressants inhibit the norepinephrine reuptake mechanism.

thetic nervous system. Other workers identified a similar pump for serotonin, serving the same purpose. Eventually, researchers determined that all amine and amino acid neurotransmitters are inactivated after synaptic release by such pumplike systems. The mechanism of enzymatic degradation that inactivates acetylcholine turns out to be an exception to the general rule. Reuptake pumps are the standard way in which the nervous system inactivates amine and amino acid neurotransmitters after the transmitters have been released into the synapse.

Axelrod wondered whether any psychoactive drugs worked by blocking the action of this reuptake mechanism. He screened many substances, among them imipramine and related tricyclic antidepressants. These turned out to be powerful inhibitors of the norepinephrine uptake mechanism—more powerful than any of the other compounds he tested—a discovery that readily explained the therapeutic effects of the tricyclics. By inhibiting the reuptake inactivation of amine neurotransmitters, tricyclic antidepressants leave more transmitter molecules in the synaptic cleft, thus potentiating their effects upon receptor sites (see the diagram below). The end result is thus functionally similar to the potentiating effects of the monoamine oxidase inhibitors.

The Amine Hypothesis of Depression

By the early 1960s, all sorts of laboratory and clinical data had begun to coalesce into a coherent picture. All the clinically effective tricyclic antidepres-

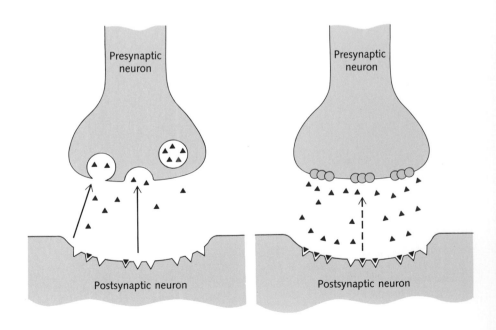

Normal reuptake inactivation of norepinephrine (*left*) and its inhibition by tricyclic drugs (*right*).

sants had been seen to inhibit the reuptake of norepinephrine and serotonin. Therefore, of the amine neurotransmitters, norepinephrine and serotonin seemed to be the best candidates for a role in antidepressant action. Several tricyclic antidepressants also inhibited the reuptake of dopamine, but as a number of clinically useful tricyclic drugs had no effect whatever upon dopamine reuptake, dopamine was eliminated from serious consideration as the key to antidepressant drug action.

At this time, researchers developed procedures to map norepinephrine and serotonin neurons in the brain. A common technique was to expose brain slices to formaldehyde vapors, which caused norepinephrine to fluoresce bright green and serotonin to appear yellow. Examination of slices prepared in this way showed that the cell bodies of norepinephrine- and serotonin-containing neurons are concentrated in discrete groups throughout the brain stem (see the illustration on page 108). The ascending axons of these neurons travel to numerous parts of the brain, but the highest density of norepinephrine- and serotonin-containing nerve endings was found in the limbic system. As we saw earlier, this is the portion of the brain that regulates emotional behavior. It therefore makes very good sense that these two neurotransmitters would influence an emotional disease like depression.

Contemporary clinical findings also supported an amine hypothesis of depression. By the end of the 1950s, chlorpromazine and related drugs were

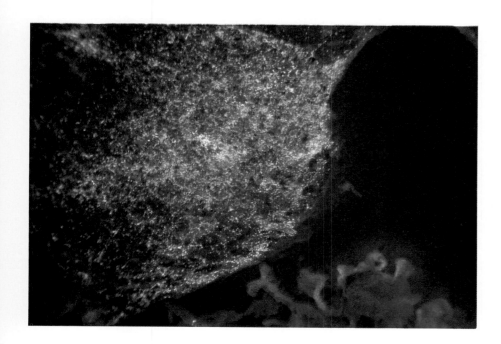

Norepinephrine neurons of the solitary tract nucleus of a rat fluoresce green when exposed to formaldehyde.

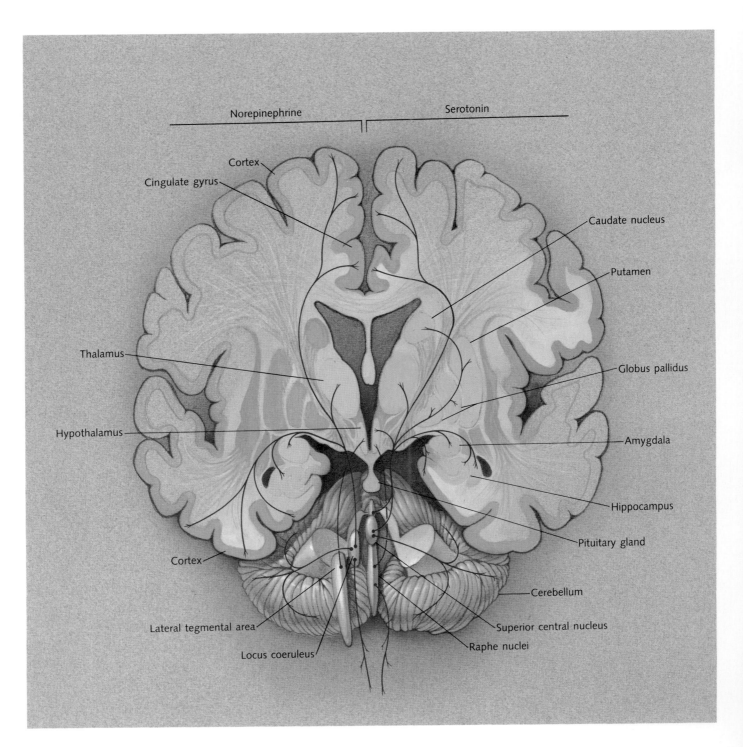

becoming the agents of choice in treating schizophrenia. Reserpine was gradually fading from use as an antischizophrenic because it caused such a marked lowering of blood pressure. This very ability was swiftly making reserpine one of the most widely selling antihypertensive drugs in America, but as millions of people with high blood pressure consumed reserpine, their physicians began to notice some frightening changes in their patients' behavior. Many patients became morose and then progressively sadder at the same time that their blood pressure fell from high, sometimes life-threatening levels to reassuringly normal values. On the basis of their physical condition, the patients should have been elated. It gradually became apparent that reserpine was precipitating severe depressive states. National attention was drawn to this circumstance when the *New England Journal of Medicine* published a report by the prestigious internist Edward Freis. A series of his reserpine-treated hypertensive patients had committed suicide; none of these unfortunate individuals had shown evidence of emotional illness before their treatment with reserpine began. Psychiatrists have since reported that at least 15 to 20 percent of reserpine-treated patients display symptoms clinically indistinguishable from those of severe depression.

The emotional change in hypertensives receiving reserpine was a dramatic validation for the use of reserpine-treated rats as an animal model of depression. Reserpine depleted brain levels of dopamine, norepinephrine, and serotonin, and it was now quite obvious that a deficiency of amine neurotransmitters could provoke a depressive mental state. Recalling how amine actions are facilitated by antidepressants—both the tricyclic type and the monoamine oxidase inhibitors—psychiatrists began to pay ever more serious attention to the hypothesis that depression is a disease caused by a deficiency of certain biogenic amines.

As scientists improved their techniques for detecting low levels of amines, they began to measure the amine concentrations in postmortem human brains. Several researchers measured levels of serotonin and norepinephrine in the brains of people who had committed suicide as a result of depression and compared them to levels in individuals of the same age who had been killed in accidents. The suicides' brains had lower levels of serotonin.

A Swedish investigator, Marie Åsberg, devised a way to look for serotonin abnormalities in living humans. She drew samples of cerebrospinal fluid from depressed patients and assayed them for levels of one of the breakdown products of serotonin. This measurement gave a better reflection of serotonin release than measuring serotonin itself, for when serotonin neurons fire more rapidly, the released serotonin is as rapidly converted into metabolic products, which therefore accumulate in higher-than-normal levels. Meanwhile, levels of serotonin within the neurons do not decline because homeostatic mechanisms stimulate the synthesis of more serotonin to replace the serotonin that has been released. In Chapter 3, we saw how a similar mechanism keeps neuronal levels of dopamine constant.

Facing page Norepinephrine pathways are represented on the left side of this painting and serotonin pathways are represented on the right. Cell bodies of the serotonin neurons are concentrated in the raphe nuclei, while norepinephrine-containing cell bodies are found in the locus coeruleus and lateral tegmental area.

Previously, other investigators had attempted without success to find changes in the levels of norepinephrine breakdown products. Åsberg, however, found that while many depressed patients had completely normal levels of serotonin breakdown products, a second group had levels that were very much lower (see the graph below). She suggested that there might exist two types of depression, one of which was associated with a deficiency of serotonin. Åsberg

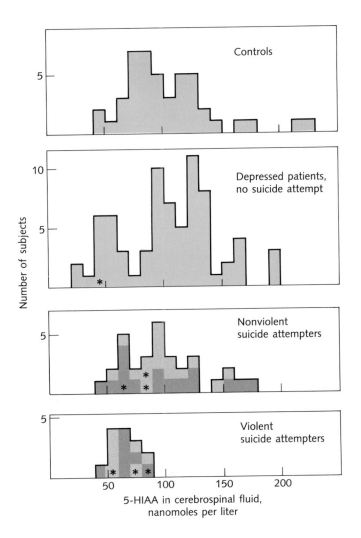

In one study, Marie Åsberg compared levels of serotonin breakdown products in the cerebrospinal fluid of four groups of subjects: normal controls, depressed patients who did not attempt suicide, subjects who attempted suicide by nonviolent means, and subjects who made violent attempts to end their own lives. (The color indicates suicide attemptors who had been diagnosed as depressed.) Those who attempted suicide had lower average levels of the serotonin metabolite 5-hydroxyindole acetic acid (5-HIAA). Asterisks represent patients who subsequently committed suicide.

tested the validity of her proposal by comparing the two patient populations on clinical grounds. The patients with low levels of serotonin breakdown products were much more apathetic and inactive and seemed to be more seriously depressed. Follow-up of the patients' progress showed that the patients with low serotonin production were far more likely to make serious suicide attempts than were the patients whose serotonin formation was normal.

Testing theories is just as important as constructing them. A good researcher develops hypotheses and then attempts, and invites others to attempt, to disprove them. Not surprisingly, research psychiatrists are continuously assaulting the amine hypothesis of affective disorders. One challenge to the theory has come from new generations of antidepressant drugs that are neither monoamine oxidase inhibitors nor blockers of amine reuptake mechanisms. The exact biochemical activities of these new groups of antidepressant drugs are unclear, but, like the earlier antidepressants, all have the ability to somehow potentiate the actions of amine neurotransmitters. Interestingly, all of the new antidepressants are also active in the time-honored "acid test" of reversing reserpine sedation in rats. Indeed, most of the new drugs were discovered through this model system.

The second-generation antidepressants also have the same clinical effect on depression as the first-generation drugs. All show the characteristic lag time of about two weeks before relief of symptoms is observed, and all influence depressive symptoms to a similar degree. The major advantage of the new drugs is the lesser incidence of side effects. Many patients experience a dry mouth, difficulty urinating, and cardiac arrhythmias as a result of treatment with tricyclic antidepressants. The new-generation antidepressants, largely free of these side effects, have made antidepressant drug therapy a less disagreeable process. This improvement is not unimportant, for the side effects of the older antidepressants are so unpleasant that many patients do not take the prescribed dose and thus respond poorly, if at all, to the treatment. From a practical clinical perspective, then, the new drugs are likely to make a marked contribution, simply because patients are more likely to take them as instructed.

The Lag-Time Enigma

The lag time of one to four weeks before depression lifts is a mystery that pharmacologists are most anxious to resolve. No one is certain of the reason for this delay in action. It seems especially puzzling when one considers that tricyclic antidepressants inhibit amine reuptake immediately and monoamine oxidase inhibitors block enzyme activity just as rapidly.

Recent evidence suggests that the delay may be required in order for the potentiated actions of amine neurotransmitters to alter the functioning of neurons in a long-lasting way. The theory runs as follows: Suppose that a neuron with receptors for norepinephrine is suddenly exposed to elevated levels of the transmitter. The neuron's homeostatic mechanisms will attempt to reduce the

Lag time in imipramine's antidepressant effect. In a typical study, a patient would be given approximately 200 milligrams of drug daily. Blood levels would reach a steady state in four days, but a definite therapeutic response might not be apparent until twelve days after initiation of therapy.

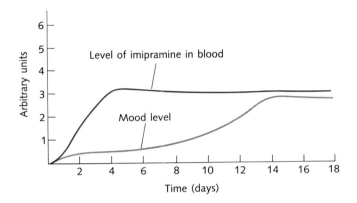

impact of the increased norepinephrine levels by instituting changes in the cell's own biochemical functioning. One way of doing this would be to reduce the neuron's actual number of norepinephrine receptors. Accordingly, the rate of synthesis of norepinephrine receptors is diminished so that after ten to thirty days they are actually fewer in number than when drug administration commenced. Scientists have measured the time that nerve cells require to alter their metabolism and reduce receptor numbers, and have found that it fits nicely with the lag period that depressed patients experience before their antidepressants exert any therapeutic effects.

Research has also shown that serotonin and norepinephrine receptors are reduced in number after chronic treatment with antidepressants, and these tests have provided the most effective means of screening for antidepressant drugs since the institution almost thirty years earlier of the reserpine-induced depression model in rats. In the new screening method, rats are treated for ten days with a candidate antidepressant drug, and then the numbers of norepinephrine and serotonin receptors in their brains are measured. Drugs that reduce the numbers of these receptors are regarded as good clinical candidates and subjected to more extensive animal and then human testing.

These new findings have introduced a novel concept into our thinking about the ways in which aberrant neurotransmitter mechanisms might give rise to mania and depression. Receptor sensitivity, usually determined by the numbers of receptors but also affected by their molecular properties, may be an important regulator of neurotransmitter actions. It is conceivable that receptors are continuously modulated in their sensitivity in normal individuals as well as in patients with mania or depression. A subtle regulatory mechanism of this type would afford evenness of mood in the face of the chaotic jumble of events that each of us encounters every day.

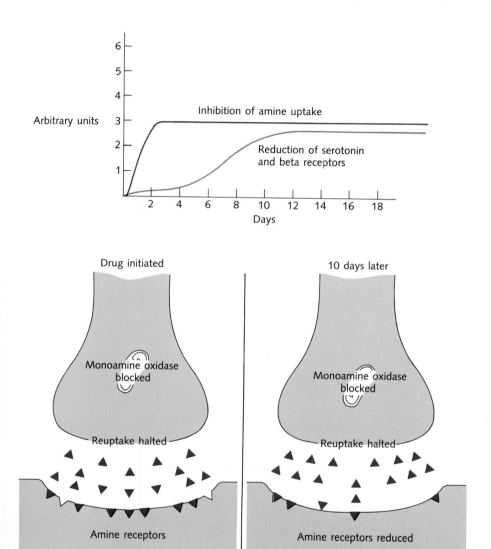

Studies of rats treated with antidepressants (typically 10 milligrams per kilogram daily) show substantial inhibition of amine reuptake after one or two days. However, a decrease in the number of amine neurotransmitter receptors is not evident until approximately ten days after drug administration begins.

Lithium, a Metal for Mania

Impressive as the actions of the antidepressants may be, the metal ion lithium has even more remarkable effects on patients with affective disorders. Not only does lithium directly relieve some forms of severe depression, but it also prevents the recurrence of depression when given prophylactically to patients who would otherwise have periodic relapses. Most remarkable of all, it exerts a direct therapeutic action on the other aspect of bipolar illness: It relieves the symptoms of mania.

The milder forms of mania can be amusing. Patients who are modestly hypomanic seem clever and charming. They manifest abundant self-confidence and boundless energy and are able to accomplish massive amounts of work cheerfully, effortlessly, and often with high-quality results. Scholars have suggested that some of the most productive figures in history were at times hypomanic—people like Winston Churchill, Abraham Lincoln, Theodore Roosevelt, and Benjamin Franklin.

Severe mania, on the other hand, is disruptive and unhealthy. Hyperactivity can become so excessive that some manic patients have been known to die of heart failure. Words and ideas follow one another in rapid succession to the point of incoherence. The patient who, when hypomanic, merely displays excessive self-confidence can become frankly delusional when in a truly manic phase. I knew such a patient, a real estate salesman, who was confident that he would win the award for having sold the most houses that year. When his manic symptoms worsened, he started talking about selling whole neighborhoods, then entire cities. Finally, he convinced himself that he could control the destiny of the world by buying and selling different countries, including the United States and Russia.

Abraham Lincoln's recurrent depressions, Winston Churchill's dramatic mood swings, and Theodore Roosevelt's constant frenetic activity suggest to historians that these men suffered from mood disorders.

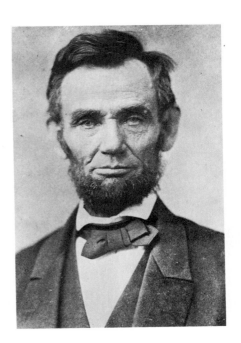
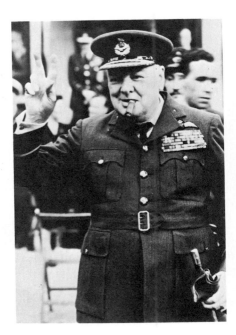
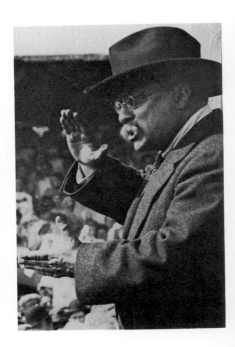

Manic patients are so frantically mercurial that small hindrances become sources of painful irritation for them. Paranoia is a typical reaction. Manics often feel that anyone interfering with their grandiose schemes must be plotting against them.

For many years, the only treatment for mania was sedation. Before the advent of neuroleptics, manics typically received large doses of barbiturates that simply rendered them unconscious. When they woke up, their manic behavior would take up where it had left off. Later, psychiatrists preferred to prescribe sedating neuroleptics, such as chlorpromazine, for their manic cases because those drugs did not put the patient to sleep, but while chlorpromazine effectively hampers a manic's activity, one can still perceive in the patient a relentless pressure of ideas striving for expression. In other words, chlorpromazine does not affect the underlying disorder. Worse yet, if a mania finally abates under treatment with neuroleptics, the patient may then plunge into a deep depression. Furthermore, as we saw in Chapter 3, neuroleptics act by blocking dopamine receptors—this is the mechanism behind their therapeutic effects in schizophrenia—and blocking dopamine receptors produces serious side effects. In the early stages of such a treatment, patients develop Parkinsonian side effects. Of greater concern is the possibility that they will later develop the irreversible neurological symptoms of tardive dyskinesia.

In contrast, the simple metal lithium, introduced to psychiatry in the mid-1960s, truly aborts the manic condition. Unlike the neuroleptics, lithium does not cause sedation; nor does it transform mania into depression. Instead, it actually seems to restore the patient to a normal state of mind.

How was such a miracle drug discovered? All the credit for this accomplishment belongs to a single individual, the Australian psychiatrist John Cade. It was his idea to administer lithium to manic patients, and the effectiveness of the drug was apparent in the very first patient he gave it to. Moreover, the dose and formulation that Cade first used continues to be the standard mode of administration to this day.

Incredibly, Cade's reasons for giving lithium to manic patients were totally misguided. While working in a small chronic psychiatric hospital in the late 1940s, Cade developed a theory that mania was caused by a toxin which, besides entering the brain, was also excreted in the urine. To test this idea, he injected guinea pigs with concentrated urine from manic patients, schizophrenic patients, and normal human controls. Each of the urine samples killed some guinea pigs, but Cade felt that the urine of manics was more toxic than the urine of schizophrenic or normal subjects.

Lacking sophisticated analytical machinery to identify the offending toxin, Cade instead injected guinea pigs with a few chemicals that are well known to be present in urine. One of the most abundant constituents of urine, urea, did indeed prove lethal when injected into guinea pigs, but urea levels in the urine of his manic patients all seemed to be quite normal. Cade wondered whether some other chemical modified the toxicity of urea and occurred in different

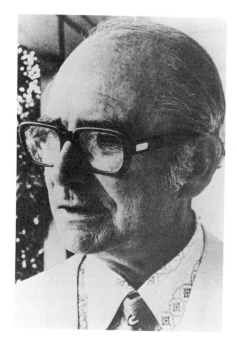

John Cade (1912–   ), the Australian psychiatrist who discovered the therapeutic effects of lithium on manic patients.

concentrations in manic and normal urine. One possibility was uric acid, another abundant urinary constituent, but when he set out to test the effects of uric acid, he encountered great difficulty dissolving it in order to inject it into the guinea pigs. He tried mixing the uric acid with a number of metals to form a more soluble salt and found lithium to be effective in this regard. When tested, the lithium urate preparation seemed to calm the guinea pigs and block the lethal effects of urea. Cade then tested lithium in another salt, lithium carbonate, to determine whether the key factor in the calming effect was the uric acid or the lithium. The lithium carbonate, too, calmed the guinea pigs. Impressed with these behavioral effects, Cade decided to administer the preparation directly to the manic patients in the wards upstairs.

We now know that there is nothing abnormal about the urine of manics. Moreover, lithium appears to calm guinea pigs only because it makes them sick. In spite of the flaws in his theory, however, Cade's clinical trial was a resounding success.

His very first manic patient was an ideal experimental subject, a fifty-one-year-old man who had been in a state of constant manic excitement for five years. Within five days, during which he took lithium three times a day, the patient's manic symptoms subsided. Unable to believe this incredible response, Cade kept his patient in the hospital for observation an additional eight weeks. Throughout this period, the patient remained perfectly well. He continued with the lithium therapy after his discharge from the hospital and commenced to enjoy a completely normal family life and a productive occupation. Cade published his findings in an Australian journal in 1949, after obtaining similarly remarkable results in another ten manic patients, but no one paid attention. The obscurity of the journal and John Cade's lack of international scientific reputation were the probable reasons for this neglect. Finally, in 1954, a Danish psychiatrist named Mogens Schou administered lithium to a series of manic patients and confirmed all of Cade's observations. Thereafter, Schou advocated lithium for the treatment of mania, and its use began to spread throughout Europe.

Even at this point, the drug was slow in catching on, especially in the United States. Drug industry economics might have been a factor. The major antischizophrenic and antidepressant drugs, introduced to psychiatry in the mid-1950s, were all patented chemical entities. This means that each drug could only be sold by the firm that held the patent, guaranteeing considerable profit to the company in question. Lithium, being a well-known metal ion, was not patentable. Thus, it is hardly surprising that the major drug companies were reluctant to spend the many millions of dollars required for toxicity studies and clinical trials before such a product could be brought to market. Not until the mid-1960s was lithium marketed commercially in the United States and abroad, finally benefitting hundreds of thousands of patients afflicted with mania. It is not clear why drug companies overcame their initial reluctance to market the drug. One factor was presumably the moral imperative to provide a

Drugs and depression

Drug	Actions
Reserpine	Depletes brain of norepinephrine and serotonin and precipitates depression.
Monoamine oxidase inhibitors	Block enzymatic destruction of norepinephrine and serotonin, elevating their brain levels and relieving depression.
Tricyclic antidepressants	Block reuptake inactivation of norepinephrine and serotonin and relieve depression.
Second-generation antidepressants	
Fluoxetine, Citalopram, Zimelidine	Block reuptake of serotonin and relieve depression.
Bupropion, Nomifensine	Inhibit neither monoamine oxidase nor reuptake of serotonin and norepinephrine. Do reverse reserpine sedation in rats and are effective antidepressants.
Lithium	Relieves mania and some forms of depression and prevents recurrences of both mania and depression. Mechanism of action unknown.

medication known to alleviate a serious illness. In any event, although lithium is not a major money maker, it is nevertheless a profitable product for the companies that market it.

In 1967, Mogens Schou made another important clinical finding. For several years he had monitored the effects of lithium on two groups of patients, one group with bipolar and the other with unipolar affective disease. All these patients were people who in the past had experienced many episodes of depression; the bipolar patients had gone through several manic episodes, as well. After years of being treated with lithium on a regular basis, most of these patients experienced no further episodes of either depression or mania. In other words, prophylactic treatment with lithium was seen to prevent depressive and manic episodes in 70 to 80 percent of bipolar and unipolar patients. To have such an effect, lithium must be acting, in some extraordinary way, on the basic causal mechanism of affective disease. It is easy to conceptualize how

Radius of lithium ion compared to radii of some ions normally found in the body.

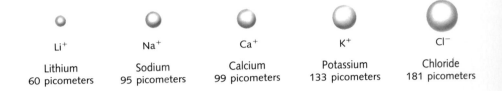

Li⁺	Na⁺	Ca⁺	K⁺	Cl⁻
Lithium	Sodium	Calcium	Potassium	Chloride
60 picometers	95 picometers	99 picometers	133 picometers	181 picometers

a psychically energizing drug might lift the mood of a depressed patient or how a sedating drug might bludgeon a manic's hyperexcitement down to a more normal level. However, for a drug to prevent the occurrence of both mania and depression, as lithium does, must mean that it is influencing some mechanism fundamental to the regulation of the entire affective system of the brain.

The prophylactic effect of lithium in bipolar as well as unipolar illness emphasizes the intimate relationship between mania and depression. It is as if our mood were normally regulated by some chemical oscillator system. In patients with affective disturbances, the oscillator is unstable and wobbles too far in one direction or another, resulting in either mania or depression. Whether the abnormal oscillations cause the system to tip more often to the "bottom" side, resulting in recurrent, unipolar depression, or whether they cause the system to seesaw from top to bottom and back to the top, causing bipolar illness, might vary with the patient's genetic constitution. This would explain the fact that in certain families one observes a preponderance of one type of depressive illness or another. Somehow lithium acts to stabilize the oscillator, holding it balanced at a "normal" level.

Of course, even though this description does fit with what we know about bipolar illness, it should be emphasized that the existence of such an oscillator is only speculative. If such an oscillating system does exist, the fact that amine neurotransmitters have something to do with affective state may tell us something about the oscillator's nature. Therefore, the next step in this line of research is to determine whether or not lithium acts upon norepinephrine and serotonin. Unfortunately, lithium is not one of an extensive series of agents, some of which are potent, some weak, and others intermediate in activity. With the neuroleptics, as we saw in Chapter 3, scientists had twenty or thirty drugs they could examine for correlations between antischizophrenic potencies and specific biochemical effects. As yet, there is no other drug that acts like lithium, and when lithium is administered to animals, it induces all sorts of biochemical changes. Chemically, lithium resembles sodium; therefore, it is capable of disrupting the biochemical systems that are dependent upon sodium, and these include almost every biochemical system in the body. At present, scientists have no idea which, if any, of lithium's dozens of known biochemical effects explains its extraordinary influence upon mood.

The interplay of science, serendipity, and sheer blunder in the development of the mood-modifying and other psychoactive drugs may perplex and alarm some readers. Science is too often described as unfolding in a systematic, sequential fashion, presided over by seemingly prescient researchers who plan every move with consummate precision, clear logic, and few false steps. In fact, this is rarely the case. One of the fascinations of the discovery process is that we often find the right answer by looking in the wrong place. The true lesson to be learned from past scientific discoveries is, "Prepare for the unexpected": be alert to chance findings, concentrate on events that strike you as peculiar, and stay hot on the trail of anything unexpected or unexplained. While these admonitions hold for all the sciences, no matter how sophisticated and well established, they are all the more paramount as guides to exploring the uncharted human mind. In the next chapter, we will enlarge our understanding of the physiological basis for moods and emotions by examining stimulant drugs, such as cocaine and the amphetamines. Their stories, too, are fraught with disappointed expectations and lucky accidents, human tragedy and a slow accumulation of knowledge and insight.

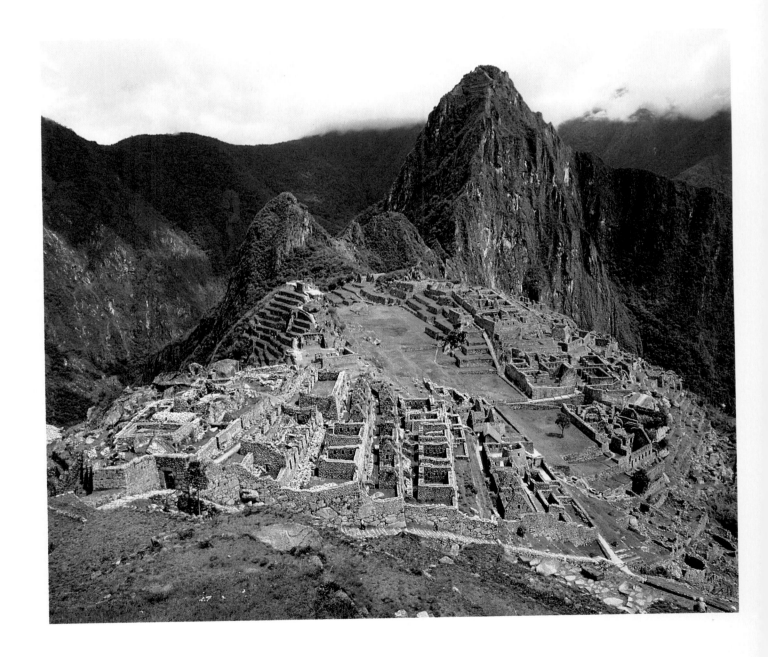

5 | Stimulants

In every culture and every age, humans have had to distinguish the beneficial applications of psychoactive substances from the destructive and undesirable ones. This has been especially true for agents that have important medical applications but that have also come to be used for recreational purposes. Many of the chemical substances used for relaxation, socializing, self-discovery, and escape are highly likely to be abused and highly dangerous when abuse occurs. As we saw earlier, opium was one of Western civilization's first medicines and also one of its earliest abused intoxicants. Cocaine and the amphetamines, which we will examine in this chapter, are the principal stimulants in the Western world today and consummate examples of drugs whose actions demonstrate both legitimate therapeutic utility and an ominous potential for abuse.

Stimulants are drugs that have an alerting effect. They improve the mood and quicken the intellect, and can therefore be valuable means of increasing mental performance and conceivably of relieving depression. Unfortunately, they are highly liable to abuse because of the dependence that users develop upon the mood-enhancing effects of the drugs. Stimulants vary in the subtleties of their effects. Caffeine, for example, does not cause nearly as much euphoria as amphetamines or cocaine. In the early twentieth century, strychnine was widely marketed as a stimulant that did not cause much euphoria. It vanished from clinical use, however, when physicians recognized its propensity to cause convulsions in doses only slightly above those that were therapeutic.

In terms of their effects on the brain, cocaine and the amphetamines are virtually indistinguishable. Any differences in effects reported by people using the two drugs only reflect differences in rate of entry into the brain related to the mode of use. For example, inhaled cocaine acts more rapidly than orally ingested amphetamine. Both are agents that increase alertness and suppress appetite. We usually think of cocaine and amphetamine as being quite distinct,

Facing page Machu Picchu, an Inca ruin high in the Andes. The Incas were acclimatized to high altitudes, but the use of cocaine made it easier for them to accomplish strenuous work under such demanding conditions.

121

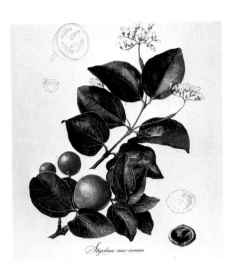

Strychnos nux vomica, source of the poison strychnine, which in the past was used in small amounts as a central nervous system stimulant.

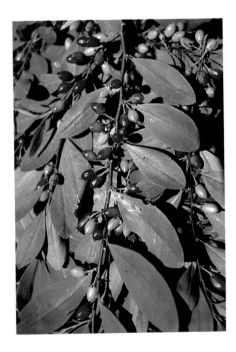

A coca shrub, whose leaves are the source of cocaine.

but that is largely because of the very different ways they entered our culture. Cocaine is primarily regarded as a recreational agent, in spite of the fact that it has definite therapeutic utility as a local anesthetic. Conversely, amphetamines were originally synthesized as therapeutic agents, and only subsequently were they discovered to have mood-altering abilities that made them attractive candidates for abuse.

Because they are so easily abused, their utilization for legitimate therapeutic purposes is on the wane. For this reason, I suspect that both these drugs will make their most positive contributions as laboratory tools for learning how the brain regulates mood. Scientists have a clearer idea of how amphetamines exert their effects than is the case for virtually any other psychoactive substance, and the same is true to a lesser extent for cocaine. In fact, the actions of amphetamines upon specific neurotransmitters have been so well characterized that amphetamine and its derivatives are routinely employed as chemical probes to analyze brain function. Much of our understanding about the systems that regulate mental alertness and feelings of sadness and joy derive from experiments that make use of amphetamines.

The stimulants' seemingly miraculous ability to enhance alertness, improve mood, and, at least subjectively, increase muscular strength has been discovered and rediscovered in different places and different times. These agents have in the past been touted as the key to health, happiness, and productivity for all. Now, their widespread use—especially of cocaine—has come to constitute a serious threat to individual and social well-being. Before delving into the chemical changes that stimulants exert in the brain, let us trace some of the events that brought these substances to their present ambiguous status in our society.

The Cocaine Story

Cocaine, labeled the drug of the 1980s because of its extensive recreational use in this decade, is also the most expensive illicit substance on the drug market today. According to National Institute of Drug Abuse estimates, cocaine is used at least once a month by four million adults and adolescents in this country, who spend a total of about $39 billion for the drug each year. Much of the drug enters the United States through Miami, Florida, where money from the sale of cocaine is laundered through city banks and accounts for a major portion of the city's finances.

Because of its sudden surge in notoriety, the drug may seem to have burst upon the United States out of a vacuum at some point in the late 1970s. This is not so. The pure chemical cocaine has been with us as an agent of abuse for over a century, and coca leaves, the source of cocaine, have been ingested for their psychoactive effects for at least a thousand years. The leaves produce essentially the same mental effects as the pure chemical, but because the leaves are chewed, the cocaine within them is absorbed very gradually from the stomach into the bloodstream, and the resulting psychoactive effects are therefore more gradual and less intense than those of the crystalline powder, which is usually inhaled or injected.

The Inca civilization of Peru accorded a prominent position to coca. Its earliest use in Inca society was confined to the royal classes and priesthood. The leaves were considered a symbol of divinity, a gift bestowed by the sun god upon the first Inca ruler. This tradition indicates that the Incas imputed remarkable properties to the plant. Clearly appreciating its pharmacological effects, they claimed that "God's angels had presented man with the coca leaf to satisfy the hungry, provide the weary and fainting with new vigor, and cause the unhappy to forget their miseries."

Over time, the Peruvian commoners became the major consumers of coca, a transition that accelerated following the Spanish invasion of Peru by Francisco Pizarro in 1533. Spanish chroniclers were greatly impressed by the effects of the leaf upon the Indians, commenting, "This herb is so nutritious and invigorating that the Indians labor whole days without anything else, and on the want of it they find a decay in their strength." Accordingly, Spanish taskmasters encouraged its use by their Indian subjects. Coca probably deserves partial credit for the incredible accomplishments of these Indians working in gold mines at high altitudes in the mountains.

Not until the mid-nineteenth century did coca leaves begin to enter Europe in substantial quantity. One of the first Europeans to popularize coca was the Italian neurologist Paolo Mantegazza, who published a widely read essay in 1859. Mantegazza ingested coca leaves himself and administered them to many others. He was impressed by the remarkable sensations the leaves induced: a general exultation, increased muscular strength (this has yet to be proved by objective measurements), a feeling of agility, smoothly flowing ideas, and an exquisitely pleasant alertness.

The dissemination of coca throughout Europe and then the United States owes even more to a Corsican chemist named Angelo Mariani. In 1863 he patented Vin Mariani, a coca extract in wine that soon became Europe's most popular beverage. In promoting his invention, Mariani blurred the distinction between a pleasantly intoxicating beverage and a medically useful tonic. Advertisements emphasized both how Vin Mariani would lift the spirits of the depressed and how it simply tasted and felt delightful. Physicians published medical articles recommending Vin Mariani for any number of common complaints, ranging from sore throat to dyspepsia. For developing Vin Mariani, as well as coca lozenges and coca tea, Mariani was lauded as one of the great citizens of Europe and presented with a special medal of appreciation by the Pope.

Mariani preparations provided the inspiration for the work of John Pemberton, the Georgia pharmacist who in 1886 designed Coca-Cola. The evolution of Coca-Cola provides an even more striking illustration of the muddy border between a pleasurable beverage and a medication. Being a pharmacist, Pemberton initially sold Coca-Cola as a headache remedy and a stimulant. In regis-

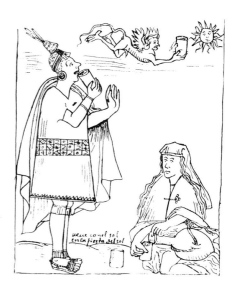

This woodcut depicts the Inca sun festival. Cocaine was considered a gift of the sun god.

Late nineteenth century advertisement for Vin Mariani. The product is described both as a soda fountain refreshment and a treatment for consumption.

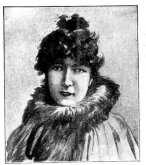

VIN MARIANI,

Mariani Wine, gives power to the brain, strength and elasticity to the muscles and richness to the blood. It is a promoter of good health and longevity. It makes the old young, keeps the young strong. Mariani Wine is indorsed by more than 8,000 American physicians. It is specially recommended for General Debility, Overwork, Profound Depression and Exhaustion, Throat and Lung Diseases, Consumption and Malaria.

My health and vitality I owe to Vin Mariani; when at times unable to proceed a few drops give me new life. It is delicious. I proclaim Vin Mariani the king of all tonic wines.
SARAH BERNHARDT.

Are You Worn Out ?

TRY

VIN MARIANI

MARIANI WINE,

The World Famous Tonic
for Body and Brain.

Mariani Wine is invaluable for overworked men, delicate women and sickly children. It stimulates, strengthens and sustains the system, and braces body and brain.

VIN MARIANI AT THE SODA FOUNTAIN.

A most refreshing, cooling, and at same time strengthening, drink is Vin Mariani taken with carbonic or soda water. Specially recommended to overworked business men, ladies when shopping, brainworkers, and all who are debilitated. It overcomes lassitude, and is helpful in the many summer complaints.

Vin Mariani taken with chipped or scraped ice is also most refreshing, and renders beneficial aid in exhaustion during hot or debilitating weather.

SPECIAL OFFER:—To those who will kindly write, mentioning this publication, to MARIANI & CO., 52 West 15th Street, New York City, will be sent, free, book containing portraits with indorsements of Emperors. Empress, Princes, Cardinals, Archbishops and other distinguished personages indorsing Vin Mariani.

Paris: 41 Boulevard Haussmann.   London: 83 Mortimer Street.
Montreal: 87 St. James St.

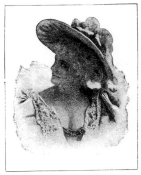

Vin Mariani is certainly unexcelled as the most effective and at the same time, pleasant tonic.
ADA REHAN.

tering the trademark, he described the beverage as "French wine of coca, ideal tonic," an acknowledgment of his debt to Mariani.

Pemberton's original preparation contained an alcoholic wine, but this was later removed and substituted with kola nut extract, a source of caffeine. The new formulation of Coca-Cola was advertised as "the intellectual beverage and temperance drink." In 1888, Pemberton substituted the base of ordinary water with soda water. Except for the fact that it still contained cocaine, the product had evolved to its present "Classic" form.

Another pharmacist, Asa Candler, purchased the rights to the drink from Pemberton and founded the Coca-Cola Company in 1892. The ensuing widespread distribution of Coca-Cola gave rise to the soda fountain as a major fixture of American drug stores, another example of the link between the pursuit of health and the quest for pleasure in Western society. Early in the twentieth century, the medical public began to appreciate the addictive dangers of cocaine (we will see why below). Eventually, the drug was eliminated from the Coca-Cola recipe and replaced with increased amounts of caffeine.

The Isolation of Pure Cocaine

Historians of the drug culture have explored the early use of the coca leaf and its extracts in South America and Europe and have found very little evidence of

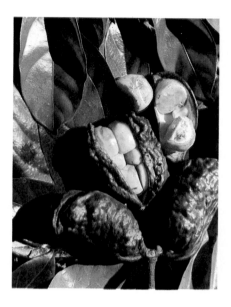

The caffeine-containing seeds of the *Cola nitida* tree.

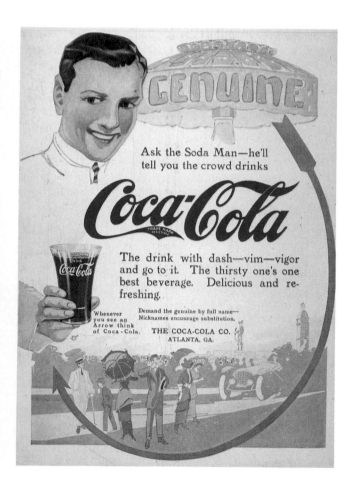

This 1914 advertisement for Coca-Cola emphasizes the beverage's stimulating effects.

abuse. Troubles seemed to commence with the availability of chemically pure cocaine. Differences in the effects of pure drug preparations and crude plant extracts have been noted with other drugs, as well. For instance, although crude opium is addicting, severe disruption of life through intense opiate addiction rarely occurred before the advent of pure morphine and heroin and their use by injection.

The middle of the nineteenth century was a period of major discovery in organic chemistry, especially in the isolation of pure chemical substances from crude plant extracts. In 1860, the German chemist Albert Niemann obtained pure cocaine from Peruvian coca leaves by mixing the aqueous plant juices into organic solvents. Cocaine would enter the organic solvent, while many of the other chemical substances, soluble only in water, remained behind in the water phase of the mixture. By performing a series of extractions with different chemical solvents, Niemann ultimately obtained pure chemical cocaine. Within two years another chemist, Wilhelm Lossen, worked out its chemical formula.

The availability of a pure chemical substance greatly facilitates scientific and medical research. Crude extracts are likely to contain a variety of substances, and one can never tell whether a plant's effects are due to a single chemical or to several. Experiments with the various chemicals isolated from coca plant extracts showed that most of the psychoactive effects of coca leaves can be attributed to cocaine: however, other chemicals in the leaves also influence the body, altering intestinal function and perhaps having some modest psychological effects as well.

Among the earliest medical investigators of pure cocaine was Sigmund Freud, best known as the father of psychoanalysis. In 1884, Freud was a young neurologist in Vienna, admired for his basic research in neuroanatomy and beginning to establish for himself a clinical practice of neurology. Freud had read about the effects of coca leaves on Peruvian Indians and also about the isolation of pure cocaine. Interested in determining whether the stimulant effects could be useful for treating nervous exhaustion, he obtained samples of cocaine from the Merck Drug Company and ingested them himself. He quickly discovered the sensations that had been known to South American Indians for millenia: feelings of euphoria, alertness, energy, and lack of appetite for food. Freud wrote his fiancée, Martha, "Woe to you my princess when I come. I will kiss you quite red and feed you until you are plump. And if you are forward, you shall see who is the stronger, a gentle little girl who doesn't eat enough or a big wild man who has cocaine in his body."

Freud conducted a number of experimental studies on cocaine. Utilizing a simple mechanical device, he demonstrated the apparent increased muscular strength produced by the drug. After evaluating its effects in numerous subjects, Freud wrote an article for the medical literature entitled "On Cocaine," in which he shared his enthusiasm for the remarkable substance with the European medical community. The publication of this article initiated widespread

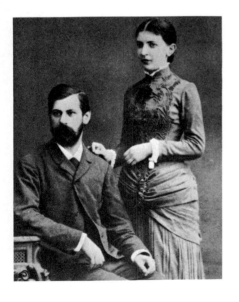

Sigmund Freud (1856–1939) and his fiancée, Martha Bernays. This photograph was taken around the time when Freud was writing his enthusiastic description of cocaine.

On Cocaine

From "Über Coca," by Sigmund Freud, July 1884:

. . . There is ample evidence that Indians under the influence of coca can withstand exceptional hardships and perform heavy labor, without requiring proper nourishment during that time. . . . [By] using coca the Indians are able to travel on foot for hundreds of hours and run faster than horses without showing signs of fatigue.

. . . A few minutes after taking cocaine, one experiences a sudden exhilaration and feeling of lightness. One feels a certain furriness on the lips and palate, followed by a feeling of warmth in the same areas; if one now drinks cold water, it feels warm on the lips and cold in the throat. On other occasions the predominant feeling is a rather pleasant coolness in the mouth and throat.

During this first trial I experienced a short period of toxic effects, which did not recur in subsequent experiments. Breathing became slower and deeper and I felt tired and sleepy; I yawned frequently and felt somewhat dull. After a few minutes the actual cocaine euphoria began, introduced by repeated cooling eructation. Immediately after taking the cocaine I noticed a slight slackening of the pulse and later a moderate increase.

. . . I have tested this effect of coca, which wards off hunger, sleep, and fatigue and steels one to intellectual effort, some dozen times on myself; I had no opportunity to engage in physical work.

. . . The main use of coca will undoubtedly remain that which the Indians have made of it for centuries: it is of value in all cases where the primary aim is to increase the physical capacity of the body for a given short period of time and to hold strength in reserve to meet further demands—especially when outward circumstances exclude the possibility of obtaining the rest and nourishment normally necessary for great exertion. Such situations arise in wartime, on journeys, during mountain climbing and other expeditions, etc.—indeed, they are situations in which the alcoholic stimulants are also generally recognized as being of value. Coca is a far more potent and far less harmful stimulant than alcohol, and its widespread utilization is hindered at present only by its high cost.

. . . Cocaine and its salts have a marked anesthetizing effect when brought in contact with the skin and mucous membrane in concentrated solution; this property suggests its occasional use as a local anesthetic, especially in connection with affections of the mucous membrane . . . Indeed, the anesthetizing properties of cocaine should make it suitable for a good many further applications.

Paraphernalia for testing, weighing, grinding, and inhaling cocaine.

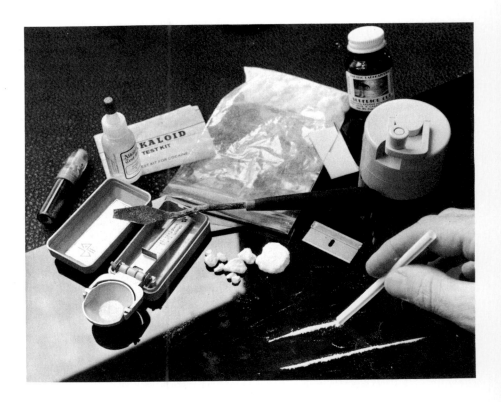

prescribing of cocaine for the relief of anxiety and depression. In the late 1800s, cocaine came to be as widely dispensed as Valium is today.

In his summary of cocaine's psychoactive effects, Freud stated that "Cocaine brings about an exhilaration and lasting euphoria which in no way differs from the normal euphoria of the healthy person. . . . You perceive an increase of self control and possess more vitality and capacity for work. . . . In other words you are simply normal, and it is soon hard to believe that you are under the influence of any drug. . . . Long intensive mental or physical work is performed without any fatigue. . . . This result is enjoyed without any of the unpleasant after effects that follow exhilaration brought about by alcohol."

A personal tragedy soon belied these initial impressions. One of the uses for which Freud had recommended cocaine was to relieve morphine addiction. A close friend of his, a pathologist named Ernst Fleischl von Marxow, had developed excruciating pain following amputation of his thumb. Though morphine relieved the pain, Fleischl became a morphine addict. In 1884, Freud substituted cocaine for morphine. Apparently, the euphoric effects of cocaine helped Fleischl withdraw from morphine, but soon he required larger and larger doses of cocaine. At this point, he was injecting himself with cocaine, a method that provided a prompt but brief euphoria followed by a sudden "crash" into severe depression. Fleischl continued to use progressively higher doses of cocaine. Finally, he became frankly psychotic, one of the earliest recorded cases of cocaine psychosis. The reason for this reaction will be discussed in detail below.

The sad experience of Fleischl was repeated throughout Europe. The enthusiasm of the medical community turned sour, and Freud was harshly criticized by all the medical authorities of Europe. The eminent German physician Albrecht Erlenmeyer denounced cocaine as the "third scourge of mankind," in league with alcohol and morphine.

Yet in spite of the inherent dangers of abuse, cocaine must nevertheless be considered one of the important discoveries of modern medicine. Most notably, cocaine was the first effective local anesthetic for use in minor surgery. General anesthesia had been introduced by the late 1840s, but it was unsatisfactory for certain types of operations. Ophthalmologic surgery is one example: general anesthesia works by putting the patient to sleep, and people's eyes move constantly in such a state of unconsciousness. Delicate operations on the

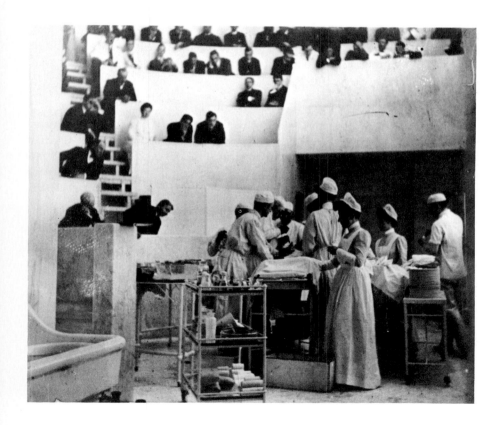

William Halsted (1852–1922) in the operating theater at Johns Hopkins.

Cocaine

Procaine

Lidocaine

Tetracaine

Chemical structures of cocaine and the local anesthetics derived from it.

eyeball therefore require that the patient be awake and able to follow instructions from the surgeon. William Halsted, the first chief of surgery at Johns Hopkins Hospital, invented local, or nerve-block, anesthesia. His approach, to inject cocaine into peripheral nerves, is still commonly employed today. Cocaine anesthetizes by blocking the conduction of nerve fibers that transmit sensation.

Local anesthesia is safer than general anesthesia and often preferable in minor surgical procedures. Much of modern eye and dental surgery would not be possible without it. Freud came exquisitely close to making the key observation himself. When he first ingested cocaine, Freud detected a numbness of his tongue and wondered whether it might reflect a medically useful anesthesia. According to his own accounts, Freud mentioned this possibility to his medical colleague Karl Koller, who then experimented with the effect of applying cocaine to the mucous membranes of the eyes. In 1884, the same year that Freud published his notorious essay, Koller reported to the German ophthalmological society the first demonstration of local anesthesia and the birth of modern eye surgery.

The success of cocaine as a local anesthetic stimulated chemists to develop derivatives that could be readily synthesized, so that drug companies could avoid the expense of importing coca leaves and then extracting the cocaine from their juices. In 1905, procaine was introduced as a cocainelike local anesthetic that produces less mental stimulation in the patient. Procaine and its derivatives continue to this day to be the mainstay of local anesthesia.

The Genesis of Amphetamine Abuse

While cocaine was first used on a massive scale for recreational purposes, amphetamine was developed with a definite therapeutic intent, the relief of asthmatic symptoms. Since the early 1900s, one of the most effective treatments for asthma had been epinephrine, also called adrenaline, the hormone secreted from the adrenal gland in response to acute stress. Epinephrine secretion is part of the "fight or flight" response of mammals, including humans, to threats in the environment. It speeds the heart rate, increases muscular strength, and dilates the bronchial tree, permitting faster and deeper breathing. These effects enable an animal to respond rapidly to predatory threats: increased muscular strength permits the creature to run more rapidly or to do battle, but the increased muscular activity demands more oxygen, which is provided by the dilated bronchial tree; the accelerated heart rate speedily delivers this oxygenated blood to all parts of the body. It is the ability to dilate the bronchial tree that makes epinephrine an effective treatment for asthma, in which constriction of the bronchial tubes causes wheezing and difficulty breathing.

Unfortunately for asthmatics, epinephrine cannot be taken by mouth. For one thing, it is rapidly destroyed in the stomach and intestines, and for another, any amounts that do escape destruction in the digestive tract are poorly absorbed into the bloodstream. Chemists therefore sought a derivative that would be sufficiently stable and absorbable to be taken by mouth. Initial chemical synthetic approaches were not productive, however, and success was delayed until the early 1920s, when K.K. Chen, a pharmacologist working for the Lilly Drug Company in Indianapolis, Indiana, began to investigate a plant called *ma huang*. Chen's hobby was investigating ancient Chinese drug classifications. In the course of his studies, he noticed that *ma huang* (whose technical name is *Ephedra vulgaris*) was frequently described as a useful treatment for asthmatic wheezing. Chen obtained samples of the plant and confirmed that its extracts caused bronchodilation in animals. In a relatively brief period of time, Chen and other Lilly chemists isolated the active ingredient, a substance chemically similar to epinephrine, and named it ephedrine (the compounds are compared on the right, below). Because it could be administered orally, ephedrine quickly became a favored drug for the treatment of asthma. No longer did patients have to rush to an emergency room or a doctor's office for an injection whenever they began to wheeze.

The only remaining problem was the scarcity of *ma huang*. Chemists were obliged to seek a synthetic substitute for its extract, and in the course of one such investigation, Gordon Alles, working in Los Angeles in the mid-1930s, synthesized a compound he called amphetamine. Alles had in fact improved on ephedrine in a major way, for he prepared amphetamine in a volatile form that could be inhaled directly into the lungs. Under the brand name Benzedrine, amphetamine inhalers became extremely popular. There was, however, very little appreciation of the new drug's abuse potential, despite the fact that Alles himself had already detected amphetamine's stimulating and euphoria-producing effects. Benzedrine inhalers were widely marketed in the United States during the late 1930s and 1940s. They were sold as a nonprescription item, as readily available as aspirin.

The ingenuity of the drug-abusing public is great. In very short order, people had discovered they could open the inhaler and ingest its total contents orally. University psychological investigators may have inadvertently contributed to amphetamine abuse when they initiated a study to characterize amphetamine effects on psychomotor efficiency in college students. A 1937 editorial in the *Journal of the American Medical Association* says, "Tablets of [Benzedrine] were used in the Department of Psychology at the University of Minnesota for the purpose of determining its effects in mental efficiency tests. It was noted that the drug prevented sleepiness and 'pepped up' the persons who were fatigued. Apparently, this information was disseminated to the student body by word of mouth and the drug has been and still is being obtained by the students from drug stores for the purpose of avoiding sleep and fatigue when preparing for examinations." *Time* magazine in the same year warned of the dangers of Benzedrine and described increasing use by students cramming for final exams.

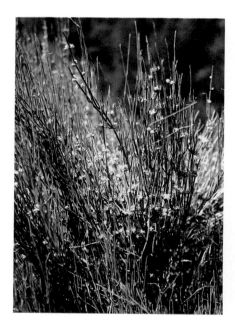

One of several ephedrine-containing species of *Ephedra*, or ma huang.

Amphetamine

Ephedrine

The apparent naïveté of the medical profession concerning the likelihood of amphetamine abuse is dramatized by reports as late as a year after the *Time* article. In 1938, two clinicians summarized their experience in the *Journal of the American Medical Association:* "There is no evidence in the entire literature of medicine that stimulants become habit forming [sic]. . . . One of us has had clinical experience with Benzedrine sulfate for more than two years in a very large number of cases and has not seen a single case of addiction."

Considerable amphetamine abuse also occurred within the armed forces of many of the countries involved in World War II. The German armed forces provided their pilots with amphetamines to keep them alert during the all-night air raids over England, and the British, too, routinely dispensed amphetamine tablets to their soldiers. Interestingly, medical consultants to the U.S. Army could not agree as to whether amphetamines were safe or dangerous, so the drugs were not officially sanctioned for use by Americans. Instead, U.S. soldiers obtained amphetamines from British army physicians. This "pass-through" was so successful that roughly 10 percent of American fighting men are thought to have used amphetamines with regularity during World War II.

Not only did the Japanese military employ amphetamines, but the drugs were systematically administered to civilians as well, in order to increase their productivity in wartime industries. After the war's end, Japanese drug companies, eager to market their massive amphetamine stockpiles, advertised the drugs for "elimination of drowsiness and repletion of the spirit." The euphoria-inducing effects of the drug appealed to many of the Japanese who had been demoralized by the disastrous war. By the late 1940s, the world's first major amphetamine epidemic was under way. In May 1948, some 1 percent of the population of the city of Kurume were found to be addicted. In fact, 5 percent of all Japanese between the ages of sixteen and twenty-five were dependent upon the drug.

Perhaps the most dramatic abuse of amphetamine occurred in San Francisco in the late 1960s. The hippies of that era, seeking to heighten the intensity of their LSD experiences, mixed the LSD with amphetamine and found that they were thus able to achieve a keener and more euphoric state of consciousness. Until this time, most amphetamine abusers had taken the drug by mouth, but members of the San Francisco drug culture discovered that routine intravenous injections provided a much more rapid onset of euphoria—followed, however, by an equally precipitous and profound state of depression. Those who injected amphetamine developed tolerance quickly and required progressively higher doses. A typical pattern of use was to take an amphetamine injection every two hours around the clock for three to six days, remaining continuously awake and excited (some of these "runs" lasted as long as twelve days). Such relentlessly compulsive self-administration stemmed in part from the fact that as soon as blood levels of the drug declined, the user plunged into a devastating and intolerable depression. Eventually, exhausted and confused, the user would fall into a sleep so deep it might last three or four days. Once awake, the

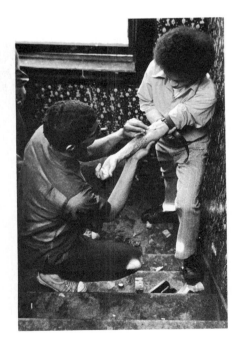

Amphetamine has been widely abused. It is most dangerous when injected, a mode of administration that provides the user with a sudden "flash" or "rush" of euphoria.

user would be ravenously hungry, having hardly eaten throughout the drug run. Apparent normality would ensue for three or four days, and then the cycle would begin again.

It's difficult to understand why anyone would seek out a drug whose effects are so disorganizing. Apparently, one major goal of the amphetamine addict is to obtain the brief but heady sensation that immediately follows the intravenous injection. This sudden, overwhelming feeling of pleasure, referred to as a rush, is often described as a whole-body orgasm. Once the user has built up to high doses, he or she compulsively seeks out the drug in order to avoid experiencing the depressive crash that is as painful as the rush is exhilarating.

The Effects of Stimulants

The chemical structures of cocaine and amphetamine are distinctly different from one another, yet for the most part their psychoactive effects are remarkably alike. Before examining how each of the drugs acts and what this tells us about brain function, then, let us briefly examine the principal mental effects that both elicit: the alertness and euphoria, the suppression of appetite, and the alarming and dangerous psychosis.

It is difficult to make an objective distinction between the enhancement of mental alertness and the increased feeling of well-being that is experienced under the influence of these stimulants. Users typically describe their euphoria in terms of the feelings of energy, power, and mental clarity brought on by the drugs. There is little doubt that these compounds bring temporary immunity from fatigue and endow the user with far greater physical and mental endurance than he or she normally exhibits.

The sense of well-being accounts for one of cocaine's earliest therapeutic indications. Sigmund Freud suffered chronically from fatigue, nervousness, and psychosomatic symptoms, such as diarrhea. In the nineteenth century this constellation of complaints was called neurasthenia. At that time, it was one of the most frequent diagnoses in psychiatry; today, we would probably label such individuals as mildly neurotic depressives. Freud was so impressed with cocaine's effect on his own neurasthenic symptoms that he recommended it as the treatment of choice for neurasthenia. When amphetamine was introduced in the United States, it, too, was recommended for neurotic depression. Although amphetamines do produce symptomatic improvement in such individuals, at least for a short period of time, tolerance to these antidepressant effects develops rapidly, and progressively higher doses are needed to produce any sense of well-being. At that point, abstinence from the drugs would produce typical withdrawal symptoms. Until recently, certain amphetamine derivatives were occasionally prescribed for mild depression, but increasing legal restrictions have interfered with such use.

While it perhaps made sense that amphetamines should ease certain kinds of depression—surely, any "upper" should alleviate "downer" symptoms—their

Actions and applications of stimulants

Drug	Effects and uses
Cocaine	Euphoria, alertness. Decrease in appetite. Used as local anesthetic.
d-Amphetamine	Euphoria, alertness, but no anesthetic actions. Decrease in appetite. Little therapeutic application except for short-term use in dieting. Used in attention deficit disorder, also called hyperactive syndrome, but decreased appetite is a side effect.
Methylphenidate (Ritalin)	Euphoria, alertness. Less appetite suppression than with d-amphetamine. Used primarily in treating attention deficit disorder.
Phenmetrazine (Preludin), diethylpropion (Tenuate), phendimetrazine (Anorex), benzphetamine (Didrex), mazindol (Sanorex)	Euphoria, alertness. Greater appetite suppression than with d-amphetamine. Used primarily for appetite suppression, but tolerance and dependence are just as disturbing as with d-amphetamine.
Fenfluramine (Pondimin)	Decrease in appetite. Drowsiness, no euphoria. Though chemically similar to amphetamines, fenfluramine's actions are different. While most amphetamines enhance synaptic effects of catecholamines, fenfluramine selectively facilitates serotonin.

effects in cases of serious depression came as something of a surprise. Experience has shown that for severe, psychotic depression amphetamines are not particularly useful and in fact tend to make the depression worse. A number of research psychiatrists have given depressed patients a single test dose of amphetamine and then a few weeks later treated the patients with standard tricyclic antidepressant drugs. In these studies, about half of the depressed patients became elated for six to twelve hours after the amphetamine dose, and the other half were immune to its effects. Subsequently, roughly half of the patients responded well to a four-week trial of antidepressant drugs, while the other patients in the study did less well. Interestingly, the patients who responded best to the antidepressants were the ones who became euphoric with the amphetamine dose. The exact reasons are unclear, but these findings do link the actions of amphetamines to the actions of antidepressants: clearly, amphetamine is influencing brain systems closely related to those affected by antidepressants (more on this topic later).

Cocaine and amphetamines both suppress the appetite, but while there is little doubt that patients treated with those stimulants initially eat less and lose weight, they become tolerant to that effect within a month. Nevertheless, appetite suppression was one of the major clinical uses of amphetamines for many years. Today, amphetamines are no longer recommended for the treatment of obesity except for very brief periods, usually only two weeks.

Of great interest to drug company scientists was the question of whether the appetite suppression had anything to do with the stimulant effects of the drugs. If it were impossible to separate suppression of appetite from inducement of alertness and euphoria, then it would be impossible to develop an appetite-suppressant drug that was free of abuse potential. Knowledge of whether the appetite-suppression effects and stimulant effects of amphetamines involved the same biochemical systems might lead to knowledge of how the two behaviors are regulated within the brain.

Following World War II, many drug company chemists attempted with at least partial success to tease apart the stimulant effects and the appetite-suppressant effects of amphetamine derivatives. Some of the drugs they developed are illustrated on page 136. Methylphenidate (Ritalin), for example, is a stimulant that reduces appetite much less than most other amphetamines. In animal studies, other drugs, too, seemed to decrease appetite and at the same time show a lesser propensity to cause stimulation. Among these specialized "diet pills" were agents such as phenmetrazine (Preludin), diethylpropion (Tenuate), and phendimetrazine (Anorex). However, while animal experiments differentiated central stimulant and appetite-suppressing activities of the drugs, in human studies the difference was less marked. Some drugs were able to suppress a rat's appetite with much lower doses than were needed to stimulate the rat's behavioral activity (judged in terms of the animal's motor activity within the cage). In contrast, it was hard to find doses that reduced food consumption in humans without causing behavioral stimulation as well. The government of Sweden was severely embarrassed by this subtle distinction. In the 1950s, a major epidemic of amphetamine abuse occurred in that country. The Swedish government responded by instituting strict penalties for the illicit distribution of amphetamine but did nothing to regulate the presumably innocuous amphetamine derivative phenmetrazine, which was sold there as an appe-

Chemical structures of amphetamines. All are appetite suppressants except methylphenidate, which is a relatively pure stimulant used to treat hyperactive children.

tite suppressant. The subsequent epidemic of phenmetrazine abuse was far more extensive than the initial problems with amphetamine had been.

Recently developed appetite-suppressing agents have shown that appetite suppression and mental stimulation *can* be separated in humans. Fenfluramine (Pondimin), an amphetamine derivative, is highly effective in promoting weight loss but produces no stimulation at all. In fact, it makes people sleepy. Surprisingly, this relatively safe weight-reduction medication has met with little commercial success. It seems that dieters were attracted as much by the mood-energizing effects of the original amphetamine diet pills as by their ability to curb the appetite—and perhaps they found the mood-enhancement necessary in order to achieve a successful loss of weight.

Although amphetamines are no longer considered the drug of choice in most of their former medical applications, they remain the major treatment modality for a relatively rare condition called narcolepsy. Patients with narcolepsy spontaneously fall asleep, sometimes while standing, or even walking. Emotional excitement, which makes most people more alert, often triggers a sleeping spell in narcoleptics. When lecturing to students about this condition, I often explain, "If any of you should fall asleep while I am lecturing, that is perfectly normal. If I fall asleep, that is narcolepsy." The stimulating effects of amphetamines counteract the narcoleptic patient's tendency to fall asleep, but they certainly do not cure the condition. Unfortunately, like everyone else who takes amphetamines for extended periods, narcoleptics become tolerant to the drugs. They require ever-increasing doses in order to continue experiencing the same beneficial effects, and they develop withdrawal symptoms when drug use is interrupted.

Another of amphetamine's remaining therapeutic uses is one that at first glance presents something of a paradox. Amphetamines have a surprising ability to calm the younger victims of a condition called variously "the hyperactive syndrome," "minimal brain dysfunction," and "attention deficit disorder." These names provide clues as to the behavioral abnormalities of the condition, the most obvious of which is hyperactivity. Affected children just cannot sit still. Parents often describe the problem as commencing in the first years of a child's life: "When he was two or three years old, we were run ragged following after him, trying to get him to stay in one spot for at least a minute or two." Hyperactive children generally do poorly in school. They disrupt classroom activities by constantly moving about and becoming involved in everything but their assigned work. Teachers feel guilty about punishing these children, who are not really malicious and do not deliberately hurt others but who seem completely incapable of self-control.

If nothing is done to correct the condition, hyperactive children eventually come to think of themselves as being "stupid" and "bad." They usually have normal or above-normal intelligence, but their poor self-image can ultimately lead to failure in adult activities. A number of psychiatrists feel that the disorder continues into adulthood in some patients. Even if it does not, the poor self-image developed in childhood is likely to create problems later in life.

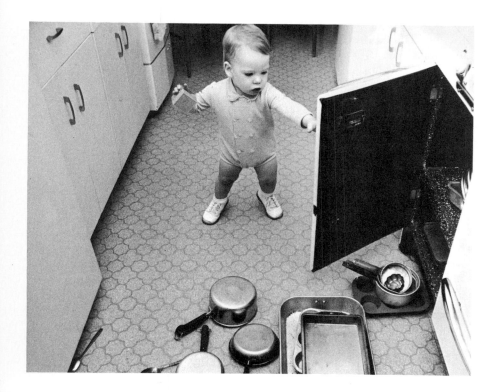

Any parent of a two-year-old might find this scene familiar, but this particular child has been diagnosed as hyperactive.

The response of hyperactive children to amphetamines is remarkable. Within three or four hours after the first dose, their behavior changes so markedly that parents are beside themselves with relief. The amphetamine-treated children become calm and even hyperconscientious. On the face of things, this pattern of effects seems categorically opposite to what amphetamines do to adults.

Careful studies by child psychiatrists indicate that amphetamines do not really calm these children down but on the contrary, act to enhance their alertness, just as occurs in adults. Apparently, hyperactivity derives from an inability to concentrate. Affected children cannot focus their attention on any one subject for a prolonged period of time. Amphetamines make the children more alert, enabling them to concentrate on one topic at a time. As a result, the young patients are finally able to keep still.

Stimulant Psychosis

Many drugs can cause frightening and dangerous mental reactions of one form or another. The psychotic states produced by cocaine and amphetamine, however, are remarkably similar to each other and quite clearly distinguishable from other types of drug-induced psychotic states. For example, alcoholics undergoing abrupt withdrawal after a prolonged binge often suffer a reaction known as delirium tremens, or "the DT's." Patients with the DT's are confused and disoriented. They do not know where they are, what time of day it is, and sometimes even *who* they are. This is an example of what psychiatrists call an "organic" psychosis, as opposed to a "functional" psychosis, like manic-depression or schizophrenia, in which patients know where they are, the time of day, and so forth. Organic psychosis can be caused by organic insults to the brain, such as brain tumors. Cocaine or amphetamine psychosis, on the other hand, is not usually accompanied by a clouding of consciousness. Instead, patients are quite alert and fully aware of who they are, where they are, the time of day, and the day of the week; in other words, stimulant psychosis is reminiscent of a functional psychosis.

Stimulant psychoses bear another resemblance to schizophrenia: the victims are plagued by auditory hallucinations, this simply means that they hear voices. Auditory hallucinations are quite typical of schizophrenia, whereas patients with toxic organic psychoses are more likely to have visual hallucinations instead. For instance, patients with delirium tremens see vivid and frightening images, strange animals fleeting by or bizarre geometric patterns.

Amphetamine psychosis most closely resembles a specific subtype of schizophrenia known as paranoid schizophrenia. Even before reaching a state of unmistakeable psychosis, cocaine and amphetamine users develop a vague suspiciousness. This gradually worsens to a point where they feel that everything going on in the environment has special relevance to them, an obsession referred to by psychiatrists as an "idea of reference." The evening news on television may report a plane crash, a rape, election results, or football scores, but the drug user is convinced that the news has unique importance and significance for him, even though he has difficulty explaining just what the significance might be. As the ideas of reference worsen, frank delusions develop. The addict comes to feel that enemies are all about, formulating malevolent plots. The only defense is to retaliate. Thus, stimulant drug users frequently arm themselves, and many deaths have resulted from the delusions of cocaine or amphetamine psychotics.

Perhaps the most important similarity between stimulant psychosis and schizophrenia is the finding that the antischizophrenic neuroleptic drugs relieve the symptoms of cocaine and amphetamine psychoses better than any other therapeutic intervention. Although these psychoses usually subside as the drugs are excreted from the body, physicians have administered a number of different agents in attempts to abort these psychotic episodes more quickly. Sedating drugs such as barbiturates and Valium have not been particularly useful; in fact, barbiturates make the psychosis worse. In contrast, the antischizophrenic neuroleptic agents, acting like specific antidotes, have been known to bring a flagrant psychotic episode to an abrupt halt. Laboratory tests show that low doses of antischizophrenic agents have the same effect on behavioral symptoms induced by cocaine and amphetamines in animals. One way drug companies have learned to screen for potential new antischizophrenic drugs is by examining each compound's ability to block the effects of amphetamines on the behavior of rats.

Yet another clue to the relationship between stimulant psychosis and schizophrenia is the effect that stimulants have on certain schizophrenic patients. When certain schizophrenics in remission are given very small doses of amphetamines, they immediately become floridly psychotic, and the psychotic symptoms brought on in these circumstances are identical to the patient's own symptoms when he or she was most severely ill. In other words, rather than superimposing some new type of psychotic disturbance upon the existing schizophrenia, amphetamines merely activate the patient's own intrinsic disorder. This worsening of symptoms does not occur in all schizophrenics, but instances of such a reaction have been observed in all subtypes of schizophrenia, nonparanoid as well as paranoid. Most remarkable about these effects is the rapidity with which they are activated by intravenous infusions of the drugs. Delusions and hallucinations have been known to appear within a minute after amphetamine administration. The specificity of these effects is apparent from studies in which the same amphetamines in the same doses have been administered to other psychiatric patients. Depressed and manic individuals do not show any pronounced change in symptomatology when treated in this way.

Thus, stimulant psychosis appears to be a sort of drug-induced schizophrenia. Nevertheless, it does differ in some ways from the classic descriptions of the disease. For example, cocaine and amphetamine psychoses are invariably paranoid, whereas only particular subsets of schizophrenia exhibit pronounced paranoid delusions. Moreover, classical schizophrenia displays a peculiar disturbance of thinking, with a "loosening" of mental associations, and many psychiatrists do not feel that stimulant drug users manifest this typical schizophrenic thought disorder—although other psychiatrists hold that stimulant users do show distinctly schizophrenic aberrations of thinking. This debate has been fueled by the fact that many patients have been admitted to psychiatric hospitals with a diagnosis of schizophrenia and sustained that diagnosis until their history of drug abuse was brought to light. Presumably, these patients were diagnosed as schizophrenics because the psychiatrist felt they had all the major symptoms of schizophrenia, including the characteristic thought disorder.

One unique type of hallucination occurs in cocaine and amphetamine psychosis but is rare in schizophrenia or any other psychotic state. This is the hallucination of touch. It begins with an itching or tingling sensation that causes patients to examine their skin and to scratch and rub it in hope of obtaining relief. Eventually, the victims formulate delusions to explain these sensations, often arguing that lice, worms, or small animals have been placed underneath their skin. Monkeys who are chronically administered large doses of amphetamine or cocaine also examine and scratch their skin, very much like their human counterparts.

These differences aside, the ability of antischizophrenic drugs to serve as antidotes to stimulant psychosis and the ability of small doses of amphetamines to activate schizophrenic symptoms suggest that some important connection does exist. An understanding of how stimulants act in the brain to elicit psychosis should therefore provide some glimmer of understanding about the nature of brain abnormalities in schizophrenia. And, in fact, research clarifying how amphetamines influence neurotransmitters has come up with interesting parallels to the effects that antischizophrenic neuroleptic drugs have on neurotransmitters, effects that we discussed in Chapter 3. Apart from what it teaches us about feelings of elation, alertness, and vigor, this research into the actions of stimulant drugs may also enhance our understanding of the molecular causes of schizophrenia.

How Stimulants Act in the Brain

When pharmacologists are asked to explain how a drug produces its effects in humans, the first thing they do is look at the drug's chemical structure and compare it with that of known neurotransmitters. This is a most logical first step because virtually all psychoactive drugs act via one neurotransmitter or another. At this point, the task of explaining the actions of cocaine and amphetamines becomes relatively easy, for the amphetamines closely resemble dopamine and norepinephrine, two major neurotransmitters contained in

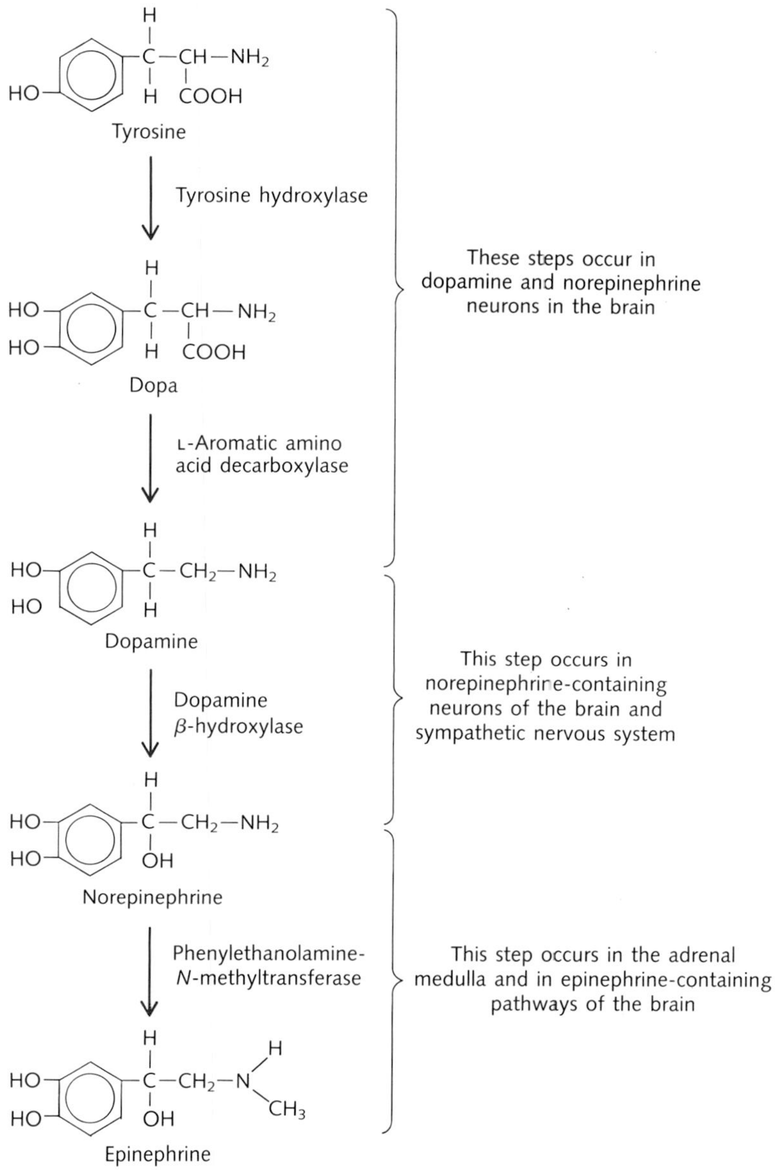

H
|
C—CH—NH$_2$
| |
HO—⬡—H COOH

Tyrosine

↓ Tyrosine hydroxylase

H
|
HO— C—CH—NH$_2$
| |
HO—⬡—H COOH

Dopa

↓ L-Aromatic amino acid decarboxylase

H
|
HO— C—CH$_2$—NH$_2$
|
HO ⬡ H

Dopamine

↓ Dopamine β-hydroxylase

H
|
HO— C—CH$_2$—NH$_2$
|
HO—⬡ OH

Norepinephrine

↓ Phenylethanolamine-N-methyltransferase

H   H
| |
HO— C—CH$_2$—N
| \
HO—⬡ OH   CH$_3$

Epinephrine

These steps occur in dopamine and norepinephrine neurons in the brain

This step occurs in norepinephrine-containing neurons of the brain and sympathetic nervous system

This step occurs in the adrenal medulla and in epinephrine-containing pathways of the brain

Steps in the enzymatic synthesis of dopamine, norepinephrine, and epinephrine.

Norepinephrine

Dopamine

Amphetamine

Facing page Norepinephrine pathways in the brain. The pathways shown in blue arise from the locus coeruleus. Those depicted in red originate in the lateral tegmental area.

brain pathways that regulate emotional behavior. In Chapter 3, when considering the actions of antischizophrenic neuroleptic drugs, we reviewed the location of the dopamine neuronal pathways. Those that seemed the most likely sites of the drugs' antischizophrenic actions were pathways that projected to the limbic, "emotional," system of the brain. Norepinephrine neurons, too, are abundant in limbic areas; however, there are a number of differences in the exact locations of norepinephrine and dopamine neurons. One of the major differences has to do with the location of the cell bodies where the neuronal pathways originate.

The bulk of the norepinephrine neurons in the brain have their origin in a very small nucleus in the brainstem called the locus coeruleus. Like many other anatomical designations, this is an imposing name with a very simple meaning. Coeruleus comes from the Latin and Greek words for the color blue. If one slices through a human brain at the level of the locus coeruleus, one sees a small blue oval.

The locus coeruleus is one of the most remarkable structures in the brain. In human brains, it contains only three thousand neurons—not a large number when one considers the several billion neuronal cells that comprise the cerebral cortex—yet from these three thousand cells arise axons that extend for vast distances and, according to some neuroanatomists, branch out to touch as many as a third to a half of all the cells in the brain. Some of the axons project upward, to the highest portions of the cerebral cortex. Others reach backward and enter the cerebellum, the part of the brain regulating fine motor coordination. Some branch in both directions, sending one axonal division to the cortex and another to the cerebellum. Along the way, each one of the three thousand locus coeruleus neurons branches profusely and makes contacts with many other brain cells. The ramifications of these cells are so vast that three thousand neurons may influence several billion.

This extraordinary situation, in which a handful of neurons affect so many others, is unmatched by any other type of nerve pathway. Until the first mapping of the norepinephrine neuronal system in the mid-1960s, most neuroanatomists assumed that neurons made discrete point-to-point contacts with only a dozen or perhaps a few hundred branchings. For a discrete cluster of cells to "touch" the entire brain was an unprecedented concept. In the early 1960s, when the Swedish researchers Kjell Fuxe and Annica Dahlström first presented these findings at international scientific meetings, the news was greeted with disbelief. Fuxe and Dahlström had employed a novel staining procedure to visualize the norepinephrine neurons, based on their discovery that norepinephrine and dopamine fluoresce bright green when exposed to an aqueous formaldehyde vapor. Their procedure was to place thin brain slices in a box whose atmosphere was adjusted to an appropriate concentration of formaldehyde vapor. When they looked at the formaldehyde-treated slices through a microscope dopamine and norepinephrine neurons could be identified by their bright green color. Additional chemical treatments made it possi-

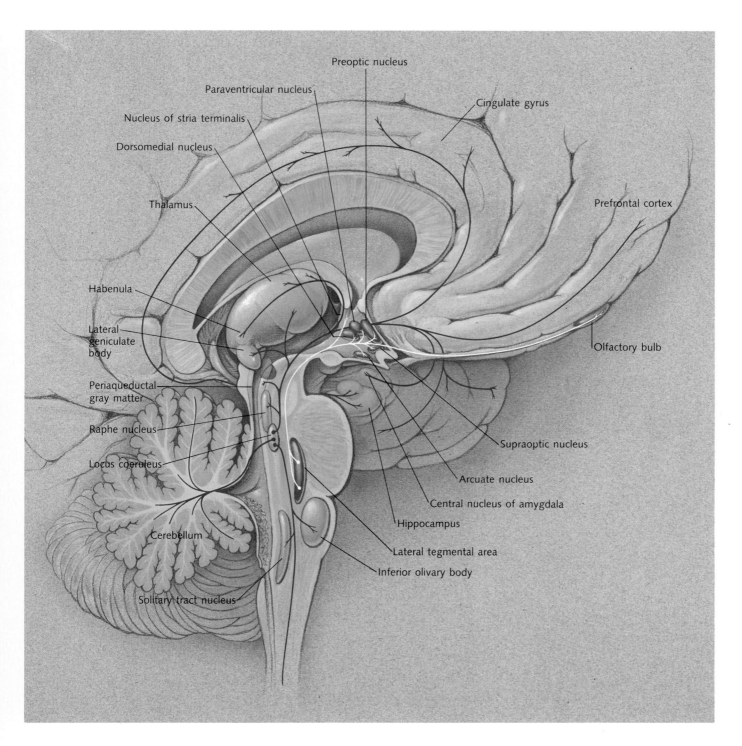

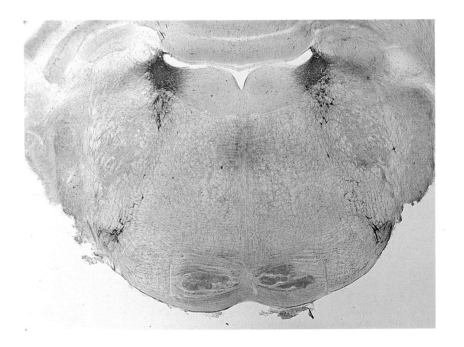

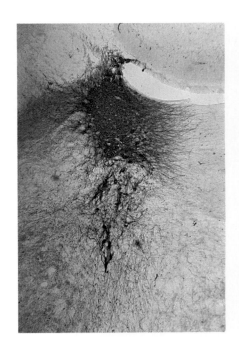

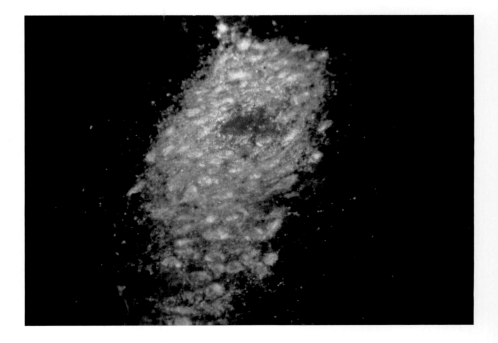

Above left Low-magnification view of a rat brain section. The two dark patches on either side near the top are the clusters of norepinephrine cells that form the locus coeruleus. *Above right* Higher magnification of one of the norepinephrine clusters visible on the left. Some of the fibers emanating from the locus coeruleus are visible.
Right Fuxe and Dahlström's technique reveals norepinephrine-containing neurons in the locus coeruleus of a rat.

ble to distinguish which neurons contained dopamine and which contained norepinephrine.

The implications of this work are considerable in terms of what it suggests about how the brain functions and how amphetamines and cocaine exert their effects. To appreciate the implications for the functioning of the norepinephrine system, let us contrast the locus coeruleus neurons with those of the visual system. When a light impulse contacts one of the rods or cones in your eye, it triggers the firing of a specific neuron that makes a point-to-point connection with another neuron in the lateral geniculate, a way station for processing visual information. From the lateral geniculate another neuron proceeds to the visual portion of the cerebral cortex. These connections are precise and unvarying and do not involve extensive branching. For this reason, we are able to gaze upon our environment and register it with cameralike precision. The neurons that account for mental processes such as mathematical manipulations

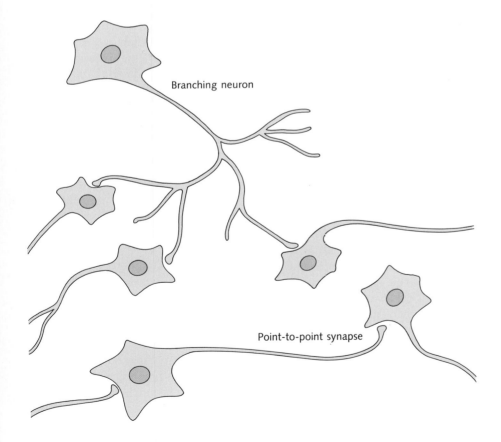

Branching neuron

Point-to-point synapse

Brain scientists theorize that logical thinking involves point-to-point neuronal connections, whereas branching connections are more likely to have a role in the generation of emotions.

must have the same type of discrete point-to-point connections, much like the wires in a computer circuit.

The very diffuse way in which norepinephrine neurons impinge in an apparently nonspecific manner upon most of the cells in the cerebral cortex is inconsistent with the idea that norepinephrine might have a role in detailed intellectual processing. In no way do the norepinephrine projections resemble the type of "hard wiring" necessary for doing multiplication and long division or other precise mental operations. However, it is possible that the norepinephrine neurons act to modulate the state of excitability of the cerebral cortex neurons that *are* responsible for detailed intellectual activity. Researchers have in fact established that the norepinephrine cells in the locus coeruleus begin firing in response to the kinds of environmental events that cause emotional stimulation, and the firing of those cells causes a release of norepinephrine at nerve endings all over the cerebral cortex. Perhaps this is how cortical neurons become "aware" of the altered feeling state of the organism. We all recognize the way our feelings "color" our thinking processes. Many brain researchers consider the norepinephrine neuronal system to be an important part of this process.

Accordingly, the norepinephrine system, with its myriad branching connections, is thought to regulate emotional responses to the environment. Any scene that we witness, be it a mother fondling her small infant or a murderer in the act of killing, is accompanied in our mind by some kind of feeling. Some emotion characterizes our every perception and thought, determining whether we find an experience to be pleasant or sad and whether an event in our vicinity will grab our attention or be disregarded. Let us examine a few of the norepinephrine pathways that emerge from the locus coeruleus and related nuclei. By knowing exactly which brain structures receive norepinephrine neurons, we can make inferences about the precise brain structures involved in generating emotional responses to the environment.

Norepinephrine neurons are more concentrated in the limbic system than in any other part of the brain. This fact alone would suggest that norepinephrine has an important role in engendering feeling states, such as love and hate, joy and sadness. One prominent group of norepinephrine neurons descends to the spinal cord, where they influence neurons that regulate the muscles of our arms and legs. There is evidence that these norepinephrine neurons play an as yet undefined role in muscle tension. Perhaps they are responsible for the physical tenseness that accompanies a mental state of vigilance and apprehension.

How, then, might amphetamines and cocaine act on the norepinephrine neurons and the dopamine neurons to make the user feel happy, alert, and energetic? Both types of stimulant enhance norepinephrine and dopamine neuronal function through one mechanism or another. Apparently, the major action of amphetamines is to release dopamine and norepinephrine from the storage vesicles (see the figure on the facing page). The amphetamine molecules diffuse into the nerve ending where the neurotransmitter is contained and, because of their close chemical similarity to dopamine and norepinephrine,

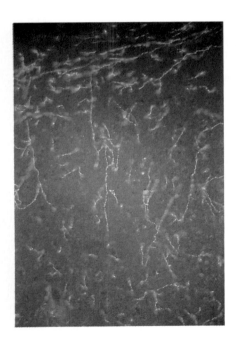

Norepinephrine neurons in the cerebral cortex of a rat. These cells were identified by means of a radioactively labeled antibody which binds to an enzyme that synthesizes norepinephrine.

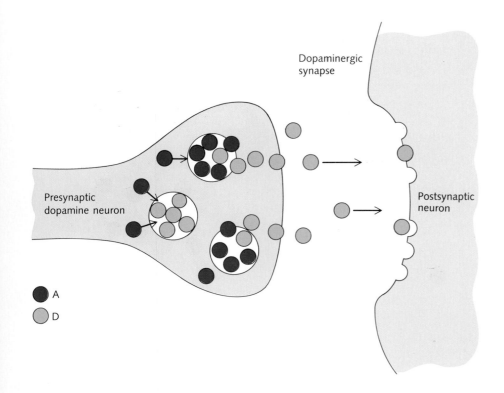

Dopaminergic synapse

Presynaptic dopamine neuron

Postsynaptic neuron

A

D

Amphetamines (A), which are structurally similar to dopamine (D), displace dopamine molecules from storage vesicles in the nerve ending, thus causing the neurotransmitter to diffuse into the synaptic gap.

displace those neurotransmitters from their storage sites. The neurotransmitters are thus pushed out into the synaptic cleft, where they stimulate appropriate receptors.

Cocaine may behave in exactly the same way, but, to date, scientists have been unable to define its precise molecular action. One thing they do know is that both cocaine and the amphetamines inhibit the pump that ordinarily inactivates norepinephrine and dopamine. This is the same action exerted by the tricyclic antidepressant drugs. As we saw in Chapter 4, after norepinephrine and dopamine have been released into the synapse, they are normally inactivated by being pumped back into the nerve endings that originally released them. Cocaine, amphetamines, and the tricyclic antidepressant drugs can all block this reuptake process, leaving greater-than-normal levels of norepinephrine or dopamine in the synaptic cleft. Researchers have tried to determine to what extent this activity is responsible for the behavioral effects of stimulants. So far, the bulk of experimental evidence suggests that, at least for amphetamines, blockage of the reuptake process is not terribly important, and that the drugs' effects are chiefly a result of amphetamines entering the neuronal endings and "pushing" the neurotransmitters out into the synaptic cleft.

Cocaine (C) prevents dopamine (D) from being reabsorbed into the presynaptic neuron. The neurotransmitter remains in the synapse, where it continues to stimulate the postsynaptic neuron. It is not known whether or not this inhibition of dopamine reuptake is cocaine's principal mechanism of action.

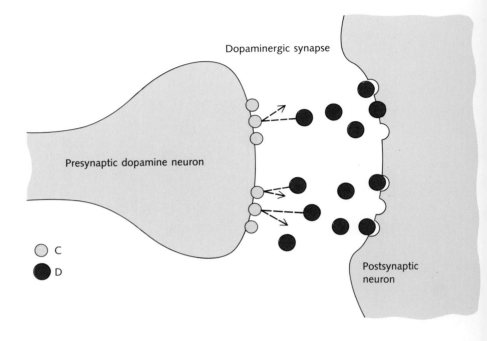

Whatever the detailed molecular mechanisms may be, the end result is quite easily explained. The alerting, stimulating effects of cocaine and amphetamines are produced by an enhancement of norepinephrine activity in the cerebral cortex. The euphoria brought on by these drugs probably involves the limbic system. The perceived increase in muscular strength and endurance can be attributed in part to enhancement of the user's mood and alertness but also to stimulation of the norepinephrine neurons that regulate muscular activity. Of course, no one asserts with absolute assurance that amphetamine, cocaine, or any other drug produces a behavioral effect via a specific neuronal mechanism. The brain is so complicated that, at this stage in our understanding, any explanation of how a drug acts involves a substantial amount of inferential reasoning. The evidence is largely circumstantial. However, the bulk of circumstantial evidence does suggest that the norepinephrine neurons in the brain have a great deal to do with the way amphetamines and cocaine increase alertness and confer a feeling of euphoria.

The answer to how amphetamines and cocaine cause a schizophrenia-like psychosis is also fairly straightforward, if highly inferential. As we discussed in Chapter 3, antischizophrenic neuroleptic drugs achieve their therapeutic effects by blocking dopamine receptors. The exacerbation of schizophrenic symptoms with small doses of amphetamines can therefore be explained by the stimulant drugs' ability to augment dopamine release. When nonschizophrenic drug users ingest progressively larger doses of amphetamines or cocaine, massive amounts of dopamine are released, and a state of schizophrenia-like psychosis is the result.

The "dopamine hypothesis" of schizophrenia, introduced in Chapter 3, grew out of the realization that amphetamine and cocaine, which can cause psychosis, and the neuroleptic drugs, which inhibit psychosis, both exert a marked effect on dopamine transmission in the brain. Of the myriad drugs that influence the mind—alcohol, barbiturates, psychedelic drugs, marijuana, and so forth—only the stimulants and the neuroleptic drugs produce mental effects that are intimately associated with the schizophrenic process; and of all the major psychoactive drugs, these exert the most selective effects upon dopamine systems in the brain. Thus, whether or not an abnormality of dopamine is central to the schizophrenic process, there is little doubt that dopamine neurons are closely related to brain processes that influence schizophrenic behavior.

Cocaine has come in recent decades to be considered one of the great scourges of humankind. As therapeutic modalities, the amphetamines, once among the most widely prescribed drugs in the United States, have fallen into disrepute. Perhaps the greatest contribution we can expect from these drugs in the future will be their utility as tools of neurological research, probes that enable us to understand some of the normal and pathological workings of the brain.

In the next chapter, we will return to the realm of psychiatry to confront an ambiguous emotional condition whose cause or causes remain a mystery, whose status as a disease is in question (in sharp contrast to what we have just learned about schizophrenia), but whose disagreeable effects are quite efficiently alleviated by a remarkable group of compounds, the benzodiazepines. We will see why these drugs have been more helpful than any others in explaining how neurotransmitters affect the rate of neuronal firing in the brain.

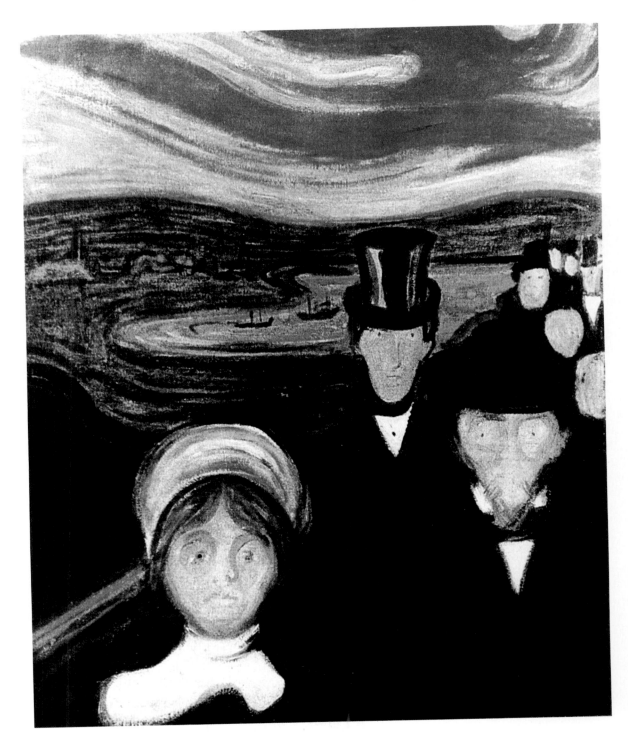

6 | Easing Anxiety

When physicians diagnose schizophrenia, they do not know whether they are dealing with a single disease entity common to all schizophrenics or with a collection of different conditions that produce fairly similar symptoms. The same is true of manic-depressive disorder. Nevertheless, most practitioners are fairly comfortable with the idea that schizophrenia and manic-depressive illness are indeed diseases. The exact causes of these disorders are not as well defined as the cause of tuberculosis or strep throat, but both conditions demonstrate some degree of clinical uniformity, evidence for a strong genetic predisposition, and hints of specific biochemical abnormalities.

Anxiety has quite a different status. Many authorities argue that, in small amounts, this unsettling feeling of apprehension and uncertainty is actually a very good thing—and, indeed, most normal people exhibit it to some degree. At the same time, extreme anxiety, while not considered a disease in itself, is looked upon as a symptom—much as fever is a symptom—that indicates the presence of some disease process. It is quite possible, however, that there also exists a subclass of individuals in whom pronounced anxiety is genetically determined and should therefore be regarded as a disease unto itself, although at present there is no scientific evidence that such a disease exists.

Those who consider anxiety to be an important force in human affairs note that people who are perfectly tranquil, unruffled by the turmoil of world events or even of their own job and home life, tend not to be particularly interesting, motivated, or creative. In contrast, interviews with world-reknowned artists, scientists, writers, and business executives consistently reveal that anxiety has provided the motivation for some of humanity's most distinguished accomplishments. When such productive and innovative individuals are asked to describe what inspired them to do the work for which they came to be recognized, they typically relate that it all began when they were feeling vaguely uneasy, dissatisfied with themselves and the world about them.

Facing page Anxiety, by Edvard Munch, 1894.

The creative breakthrough reflected an effort to change themselves and their environment, to pull their minds and emotions out of some quandary that demanded resolution.

Unfortunately, all too many people find anxiety to be a crippling obstacle that prevents them from achieving their goals. Severely anxious individuals can be terrified of interacting with others, and so preoccupied with their internal agitation that they may have trouble concentrating on work or other activity. Very extreme cases may reach a point where their life ceases to provide any pleasure, at which juncture their anxiety merges into depression and hopelessness. Because this pattern is observed in so many patients, some experts believe that anxiety mechanisms and depression mechanisms of the brain are closely related, though attempts to treat anxiety with antidepressant drugs have yielded inconclusive results. Other researchers argue that the conditions are separate and distinct but that severe anxiety is so disruptive, any reasonable person would find it a depressing experience. Sadly, such severe anxiety is remarkably common, affecting at least 5 to 10 percent of the world's population. Accordingly, whatever science and medicine can do to relieve anxious symptoms will be a boon to millions of distressed men and women.

A Clinical Picture of Anxiety

Anxiety is a broad label that can be applied to feelings of various intensities, and therefore it is difficult to define. In our exploration of the effects of drugs on anxiety, we will pay less attention to the feelings of vague dissatisfaction that affect most normal people and concentrate instead on conditions of disabling emotional distress that may lead a person to seek medical intervention.

The symptoms of severe anxiety so closely resemble abject fear and terror that we can perhaps best understand anxiety by comparing it to those sensations. In the evolution of the human species, fear, like pain, has been of great survival value because it warns the organism of danger. The body changes associated with fear enabled our evolutionary ancestors—and still enables us, in certain contexts—to deal with threatening events. Fear triggers the "fight or flight" pattern of bodily reactions that we discussed in earlier chapters. The heart rate accelerates, pumping more blood to the arms and legs and thus strengthening them to combat an attacker or to run away as fast as possible. When terrified, we breathe deeply and rapidly, and the bronchial tree of our lungs expands to facilitate the absorption of oxygen. This is because more oxygen is needed to fuel the increased volume of blood circulating throughout the body. We also perspire profusely, to dissipate the increased body heat that accompanies the augmented muscular activity.

Many psychiatrists define anxiety as a fear response in the absence of an appropriate stimulus. This hardly does justice to the excruciating suffering of patients with severe anxiety. The subjective sensation of anxiety can be much more troubling than that of fear because the source of patients' distress is so unclear, and the unknown is always more terrifying than the known. The generalized uneasiness permeating every aspect of their lives can be as difficult to endure as a constant and severe physical pain.

Anxious people almost unvariably will maintain that they have no idea why they are feeling so uncomfortable. Even after months or years of intensive psychotherapy aimed at pinpointing the source of their problem, many patients fail to uncover likely connections between feelings about father, mother, wife, or sibling and their present agony. In an almost frantic attempt to find some basis for their terror, patients will blame anything and everything in the environment: a minor setback at work, a neighbor's noisy dog, the flu, a disobedient son or daughter. Most of these efforts at justification fail to bring relief. Patients continue to complain of an inner "shakiness," extreme irritability, a sense of impending catastrophe, and a terror of everybody and everything about them. Adolescents, confronting their developing bodies and changing relations to others, tend to be anxious and show many of the typical symptoms, but teenagers usually improve greatly when they enter adulthood.

The subjective sensation of anxiety is often accompanied by symptoms of physical illness. Indeed, many victims of severe anxiety first approach their physician with physical complaints, never mentioning emotions. Cardiac complaints are probably the most frequent physical manifestations. Many anxious patients are exquisitely aware of their heartbeat, which may or may not be accelerated. They are disturbed by a heavy pounding of the heart against the chest wall, especially when they are lying on their side. This emotionally induced cardiac "overwork" often provokes symptoms reminiscent of angina, to the extent that chest pains may even radiate into an arm. What happens is that the increased contractions of the heart create a greater demand for oxygen. (Angina is the pain experienced when certain nerves in the heart begin to fire in response to a relative lack of oxygen.) A vicious circle is established as fear of an impending heart attack exacerbates the patients' anxiety and worsens the cardiac symptoms. This is a common pattern witnessed in anxious individuals. In fact, the earliest published description of anxiety neurosis was a report written in the 1860s by a U.S. military physician who thought he was dealing with a fundamental disturbance of the nerves to the heart.

In his thorough and elegant description of afflicted Civil War soldiers, Jacob Da Costa called the condition he observed in them "irritable heart." It came to be known as Da Costa's syndrome. Had Da Costa been more perspicacious, he might have focused on the fact that his patients' physical symptoms affected their entire body. Instead, he restricted his diagnosis to the cardiac features of the condition:

W. W. H. was admitted November 2, 1863 and just returned from furlough. . . . He did a good bit of hard duty with his regiment [suggestive to Da Costa that the patient's symptoms had something to do with stress]. Sometime before the battle of Fredericksburg, he had an attack of diarrhea. After the battle he was seized with

153

lancinating pains in the cardiac region, so intense that he was obliged to throw himself down upon the ground, and with palpitation. The symptoms frequently returned while on the march, were attended with dimness of vision and giddiness, and obliged him often to fall out of his company and ride in the ambulance . . . . Violent palpitations ensued upon his slightest exertion, sometimes also whilst in bed, obliging him to rise.

Because Da Costa could find no physical abnormalities in this patient and others like him, he concluded, "It seems to be most likely that the heart has become irritable, from its overactivation and frequent excitement, and that disordered innervation keeps it so."

Da Costa was certainly correct in surmising that the abnormal cardiac activity stemmed from the nervous input to the heart, but he did not realize that the abnormal activity originated in the brain. Present-day physicians know that diarrhea and giddiness occur frequently in anxious individuals. The "dimness of vision" reported by Da Costa's patient would now be interpreted as the result of excessive breathing, or hyperventilation. When individuals breathe too deeply and rapidly, they blow off carbon dioxide; this changes the acidity and ionic composition of the blood, causing numbness and tingling of the fingers, twitching of the muscles, a sensation of lightheadedness, and blurry vision. Even when patients are told to avoid hyperventilating, they have difficulty stopping, because they feel unable to suck enough air into their lungs. Sometimes this "air hunger" is so severe that the patient will wake in the middle of the night and rush to an open window to gulp deep breaths. Other common symptoms of anxiety include profuse perspiration, especially of the palms of the hands; a flushed face; and a "frog" in the throat. Patients also describe a jittery sensation in the stomach.

In some patients, a mild chronic state of anxiety is punctuated with episodic bursts of extreme terror. In these panic attacks, all the emotional and physical manifestations of anxiety emerge simultaneously, with an intensity that can be excruciating. Often there is no obvious precipitating event. Fortunately, most panic attacks subside in a few hours, but they can, and often do, last for days on end.

Sigmund Freud considered anxiety to be at the heart of all forms of neurosis. In this way, he differed from most psychiatric thinking about neurosis both in his own time and today. In contrast to the currently prevailing notion that extreme anxiety is a symptom of illness rather than an illness in itself, Freud regarded anxiety as the essential mental disease, theorizing that all other neurotic disturbances were merely symptomatic ways in which patients responded to anxiety. According to Freud's model, anxiety is so intolerable that the psyche will go to great lengths to avoid it. The outward manifestations of these efforts to combat anxiety constitute the classic symptoms of neurosis. For example, Freud believed that patients with obsessional neuroses were transferring all their anxious feelings to a single fixed thought, usually a specific, well-delimited fear. One obsession that many people experience is a concern, after leaving the house, that they have forgotten to lock the door or turn off the stove. Freud believed that people focused on clear-cut and concrete concerns such as these in order to find some relief from their free-floating distress, the most intolerable component of generalized anxiety.

The same role was played, Freud thought, by compulsions. These are repetitive acts, such as ritualistic washing of one's hands. Psychoanalysts regard compulsions as symbolic means of escaping obsessive thoughts and their underlying anxious provocations. Similarly, phobias, such as an acute fear of flying, are ways of sequestering generalized anxiety into some narrow area of one's life. Avoidance of the feared object helps keep the anxiety under control.

Treatments for Anxiety

The two most common approaches to treating any psychiatric disorders are psychotherapy on the one hand and drug therapy on the other. For severe psychotic disorders, such as schizophrenia and manic-depressive illness, drugs are the major tools for relieving symptoms. In nonpsychotic conditions, such as anxiety and other neuroses, psychotherapy and behavioral therapy are often preferred. A psychotherapist might attempt to cure anxiety by reviewing the patient's life history, hoping to uncover traumatic interpersonal relationships that may have given rise to the neurosis. Freud and subsequent psychoanalysts felt that conflicts over sexual feelings underlay many cases of anxiety. They saw anxiety as representing the effort of the patient's ego, or conscious self, to keep unacceptable impulses repressed in the unconscious. According to this formulation, the way to treat anxiety is to help the patient become aware of unconscious impulses and the mechanisms his or her psyche is employing to keep the impulses repressed. Anxiety will vanish as the unconscious is rendered conscious.

Such psychoanalytically oriented psychotherapy may help some patients with anxiety. However, in many cases patients attain superb insight into their internal conflicts but remain just as anxious as before. Critics of analytic psychotherapy maintain that the patients who become cured are patients whose anxiety would gradually have dissipated with no treatment at all. Some research studies seem to support this theory. In one, patients entering a psychotherapy clinic were either treated by a psychoanalytically oriented psychotherapist or purposely kept on the waiting list without receiving treatment. About 60 percent of the patients receiving psychotherapy improved; so did 60 percent of the patients who were left on the waiting list and received no treatment at all.

Behavior therapy offers another psychotherapeutic approach to curing anxiety. It is based on the theory that anxiety is a learned response that can also be unlearned. There are many variations of behavioral therapy. One popular strategy attempts to desensitize the patient to the state of anxiety. First, patients are taught to relax all of their muscles. Once they have achieved a state of deep relaxation, they are asked to imagine some environmental circumstance that would normally provoke mild anxiety. Imagining a situation that provokes only mild anxiety under normal circumstances will probably not provoke anxiety at all while the patient is thoroughly relaxed in the supportive atmosphere of the behavioral therapist's office. After a few repetitions of this experience in the doctor's office, patients find they can cope with mildly stressful stimuli fairly well. Next, they are instructed to imagine an event that is slightly more stressful. Little by little, patients learn to remain relaxed even when contemplating severely stressful circumstances. Gradually, they transfer this more relaxed, less fearful response to real events in the outside world.

Behavioral therapy tends to be most effective with patients whose anxiety occurs in response to relatively specific environmental stimuli. It works well with phobias—a fear of elevators, for example, or a fear of dogs. For more diffuse anxiety, behavioral therapy is less effective and psychoanalytically oriented therapy may be more useful; although adherents of each form of treatment argue that theirs is clearly the best for virtually all types of anxiety. There have been many debates and considerable research regarding the relative efficacy of these two approaches.

In actuality, more patients with anxiety are treated by general practitioners or internists than by psychiatrists, and general physicians are more likely to employ drugs than to attempt psychotherapy or behavioral techniques. In the first half of the twentieth century, physicians commonly prescribed sedating drugs, such as barbiturates, for patients who complained of anxiety. In clinical doses, sedatives quiet patients down by making them somewhat drowsy without putting them to sleep. The rationale for employing them in cases of anxiety was that their quieting action took the edge off the patient's mental state. People who are mildly sleepy are less likely to feel fearful and preoccupied.

The general actions of barbiturates are not unlike those of alcohol, which is also regarded as a sedative, but as the table on the facing page illustrates, different barbiturates have somewhat different effects. The short-acting types are employed as sleeping pills. They penetrate rapidly into the brain, causing sleep less than an hour after their consumption, and then wear off in five to eight hours so that the patient will not be drowsy the next day. The long-acting barbiturates were used to treat anxiety. Phenobarbital, a modestly sedating and long-acting barbiturate, was most widely used for this purpose. Phenobarbital enters so slowly that the patient's brain can adapt to its sedating effects and can function in a fairly alert fashion even when the drug is taken during the day. Pharmacologists never claimed that phenobarbital was dealing specifically with the brain mechanisms responsible for anxiety. Moreover, phenobarbital and the other barbiturates were known to be addictive. For these reasons, they were not administered to patients for continuous use, only for short periods of particular stress or crisis.

Barbiturate actions and uses

Action	Onset	Duration	Uses
Ultrashort	Seconds	Minutes	Intravenous anesthesia
Short	Minutes	4–8 hours	Brief hypnosis Preoperative sedation Insomnia
Intermediate	1 hour	6–8 hours	Insomnia
Long	Over 1 hour	10–12 hours	Continuous sedation Hypertension Psychoneurosis Epilepsy

The first step toward developing drugs to act selectively on anxiety mechanisms was taken during the late 1940s. True to the pattern seen repeatedly in pharmacology, the original research was not at all directed toward anxiety. Frank Berger was a Czechoslovakian pharmacologist who had fled to London during World War II. There, in 1945, he was attempting to develop synthetic antibacterial agents that would kill microorganisms resistant to penicillin. Penicillin had already saved the lives of thousands of soldiers, but it was not effective against every kind of bacteria. In fact, the only types of bacteria that responded to penicillin were species that turned black when treated with a particular stain called the Gram stain. These species are referred to as gram-positive bacteria. Unfortunately, many of the most virulent bacteria are gram-negative, and at that time there was no drug with which to fight them.

Berger screened large numbers of chemicals to see if any could be used as a drug against gram-negative bacteria. One group of compounds showed considerable promise. When Berger injected these into mice to evaluate the chemicals' safety for use in animals, the mice became temporarily paralyzed, apparently because of a massive relaxation of the muscles in their limbs. A remarkable aspect of this drug-induced condition was that, though limp and relaxed, the mice remained fully conscious and aware of their environment.

Berger thought these peculiar effects might have clinical utility in certain muscular conditions. Patients with brain strokes, for example, usually become paralyzed in a spastic fashion, with their muscles tightly contracted. Much of their inability stems from this spasticity. And patients with low back pain, whether caused by disturbances in the discs that connect the vertebrae or by other factors, owe most of their discomfort to spastic contractions of the back muscles. Clearly, muscle-relaxant drugs would help in these and other clinical conditions. Mephenesin, one of Berger's mouse relaxers, was soon being used in humans. It proved to be a highly effective muscle relaxant and continues to be employed as such to this day.

In his first publications on the effects of mephenesin in animals, Berger commented that the drug seemed to have a quieting effect on the demeanor of the animals, an effect that he referred to as "tranquilization." When the drug was being tested in humans with muscle spasm, their responses suggested that mephenesin could reduce anxiety without making the user sleepy. These tentative findings prompted Berger to seek derivatives of mephenesin that might be even more effective in treating anxiety. He discovered that the derivative he called meprobamate had an impressive calming ability: besides its muscle-relaxing actions, meprobamate dramatically attenuated the normal viciousness of laboratory monkeys. Under the trade name Miltown, meprobamate was introduced to the American public with much fanfare in April 1955—about the same time that chlorpromazine, the first antischizophrenic drug, began to be marketed in the United States.

In economic terms, meprobamate was a spectacular success. Sales soon exceeded a hundred million dollars per year, and Miltown became a household word. The drug owed its success to the perception that it differed radically from previously available barbiturate sedatives, such as phenobarbital. It was argued that Miltown produced none of the sedating effects of phenobarbital, so patients could go about their day's work fully alert. More importantly, it was emphasized that Miltown acted selectively upon brain mechanisms regulating anxiety. In contrast, phenobarbital was merely a sleeping pill that dulled the brain without addressing the fundamental chemistry of the anxious state. Furthermore, it was suggested that Miltown was far less addictive than the barbiturates.

Over the subsequent decade, extensive studies were conducted to compare the effects of meprobamate with those of barbiturates and other agents, both in animals and in humans. Unfortunately, most of the initial claims for meprobamate did not hold up under scrutiny. Measurements of the electrical activity

Mephenesin

Meprobamate

of the brain failed to show any major difference in the effects of meprobamate and barbiturates, and examination of individuals treated with the drug showed that meprobamate did cause drowsiness roughly to the same extent as phenobarbital. Finally, meprobamate was found to have addictive potential. With chronic administration, patients become tolerant, requiring larger doses in order to experience a therapeutic effect. When drug administration is abruptly halted after long usage, patients begin to suffer from withdrawal. Symptoms of withdrawal from meprobamate resemble symptoms of withdrawal from barbiturates: hyperexcitability, intense anxiety, and, sometimes, convulsions.

The Benzodiazepine Revolution

Though meprobamate turned out to be far less impressive as an antianxiety agent than its developers had hoped, it served one very important purpose. It introduced the concept of a drug agent capable of dealing selectively with anxiety. Before its development, no physician dreamed that a drug might relieve anxious symptoms without simultaneously causing sedation. The general opinion in medical circles had been that somnolence and emotional tranquility went hand in hand. The vast initial success of Miltown in the marketplace prompted the major drug companies to search for other agents that might reproduce meprobamate's presumed antianxiety effects.

The first to succeed in this effort was the Roche Drug Company in Nutley, New Jersey, where chemist Leo Sternbach synthesized Librium and Valium. These two drugs, belonging to a class called the benzodiazepines, truly merit the designation antianxiety agent. Their story provides another example of the important role of serendipity in science.

Because no one had any idea how meprobamate acted at a molecular level to exert its putative antianxiety effect, the Roche Company's strategy was to synthesize chemicals almost at random and screen them for antianxiety activity in mice and rats. The exact chemical classes to be screened were left up to the chemists. Twenty years earlier, in the 1930s, Sternbach had begun a research career in pure chemistry at the University of Cracow, Poland. On the basis of chemical investigations he had conducted then, he now developed at Roche a group of chemicals that he referred to as quinazolines. These had no chemical relationship to any known sedative, and the great majority produced no noticeable effect on laboratory animals. By the end of 1955, after working with the series for almost two years, Sternbach had failed to identify any therapeutic potential for these drugs. He didn't even bother submitting the last compound in the quinazoline series for animal testing.

A year and half later, while cleaning up his laboratory, Sternbach found the last of the quinazolines still lying in a corner. He decided to give it to Lowell Randall, Roche's head of pharmacology, who submitted the chemical to routine drug-screening tests. Two months later, Randall reported that the compound was quite active in tests that identified agents with meprobamate-like

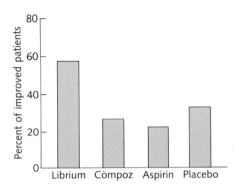

Data from a study that compared the anti-anxiety effects of over-the-counter seda-tives with those of chlordiazepoxide (Lib-rium).

effects. It was clearly more active than any of the forty other quinazolines Sternbach had developed and, in fact, was the most interesting antianxiety candidate Randall had yet encountered.

At this point, Sternbach decided to examine the chemical properties of the drug, now known as Librium, more closely. He discovered that it was not a quinazoline at all. The final steps of its synthesis had transformed it into a completely different kind of chemical, a new class that came to be called the benzodiazepines. Had Sternbach realized this in his initial synthesis, he would probably have discarded the compound, considering it a chemical error. Now, however, with an eye toward appropriating some of the massive meprobamate sales, Roche promptly put Librium through the necessary animal and human clinical research studies. By early 1960, the drug was on the market. In the meantime, Sternbach and his collaborators were synthesizing a number of Lib-rium derivatives. The most effective of these, Valium, was introduced for clini-cal use in 1963.

In developing Librium and Valium, Roche was attempting to imitate the nonsedating and nonaddicting antianxiety actions that had been attributed to meprobamate, but by the mid-1960s, psychiatric researchers were recognizing that meprobamate was not what they had assumed. Strictly speaking, the ra-tionale for developing Librium and Valium was therefore fallacious. However, as psychiatrists began to assay the psychological effects of these two benzodi-azepine drugs, they realized that, paradoxically, Librium and Valium did pos-sess many of the favorable features that had been claimed for meprobamate.

Librium and Valium do relieve anxiety. They also produce some drowsiness, but patients become tolerant to that effect in a matter of weeks and still con-tinue to obtain relief. Under the influence of benzodiazepines, the vague uneas-iness, generalized fear, and associated physical symptoms of anxiety fade away. The patient feels more relaxed and sleeps better.

Unfortunately, the benzodiazepine drugs are somewhat addicting. Toler-ance develops with continued use, and withdrawal symptoms occur when drug administration stops abruptly. However, the extent of tolerance and the sever-ity of physical withdrawal are substantially less than what is typically observed with barbiturates and meprobamate.

The most clear-cut advantage of the benzodiazepine drugs is the fact that overdoses are rarely lethal. In contrast, the lethal dose of barbiturates is only a few times greater than the dose necessary to induce sleep. For much of the twentieth century, barbiturates enjoyed the distinction of being the drugs most widely used for committing suicide. Because despondent, depressed individuals are generally insomniac as well, doctors were routinely supplying such patients with barbiturate sleeping medications. Sadly, this meant that the individuals most prone to attempt suicide were regularly provided with the most rapid and painless way of doing it. In these terms, the benzodiazepines are among the safest drugs known. Doses a thousand times greater than necessary to cause muscle relaxation and behavioral effects have been tested in laboratory animals. Mice, rats, cats, and monkeys all refuse to die. When Librium and Valium were introduced to the market, a number of suicidal patients consumed their bottle's entire contents—a hundred pills or more. They would sleep for two or three days but awaken with no apparent ill effects.

Since benzodiazepines are to some extent sedating, patients treated with Valium and Librium do not require any additional sleeping medication, even if they suffered previously from severe insomnia. All that is usually needed to transform a minimally sedating anxiety-relieving dose of the drug into a sleep-inducing dose is to take two tablets instead of one. Many patients on an antianxiety regimen routinely do this at bedtime. Some benzodiazepines are marketed predominantly for use as sleeping pills, although their general pharmacological effects are not much different from those of Valium or Librium.

As already mentioned, benzodiazepines are not totally innocuous. Their addictive potential, though milder than that of barbiturates, is nevertheless disturbing. Additionally, perhaps because benzodiazepines are somewhat sedating, they potentiate the depressive effects of alcohol and barbiturates (more on this mechanism below). When a benzodiazepine is taken with a sedative substance, the result can be lethal. Many deaths have been attributed to such a combination. Judy Garland's demise in 1969 resulted from a synergistic alcohol-Valium interaction. What is particularly disconcerting is the finding that the amount of a benzodiazepine that will be lethal when combined with alcohol is quite unpredictable and varies tremendously from person to person. Sometimes ingestion of alcohol with as little as two or three times the recommended benzodiazepine dose can halt the patient's breathing.

As physicians learned about the benefits of benzodiazepines and the drugs' apparent safety (at least as compared with barbiturates), they got into the habit of prescribing Valium with excessive liberality. In 1975, U.S. pharmacists filled a hundred million prescriptions for Valium and related drugs. Fifteen percent of the nation's inhabitants were taking benzodiazepines. At that time, Valium was the best-selling drug in the world, with total sales exceeding $500,000,000 a year. The drugs came to be used as panaceas, too often employed to relieve relatively modest distress. Many doctors prescribed them even in the absence of genuine emotional disturbance, simply to help normal men and women cope with everyday life.

Though benzodiazepines are relatively safe, such indiscriminate use is far from wise. Frank Berger himself became concerned about the abuse of benzodiazepines, as well as the abuse of meprobamate, and warned, "They are widely prescribed merely to ease problems of living. They may be effective for this purpose [only] to the extent that they dull sensibility to the knocks, annoyances and frustrations of everyday life. When used in this manner they are being used . . . not as antianxiety drugs. I find it difficult to believe that the . . . self-confidence needed to cope with one's problems can be acquired by the use of any medication."

Benzodiazepines

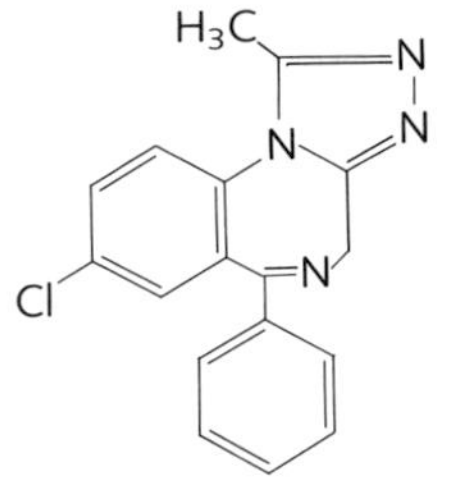

Alprazolam
(Xanax)

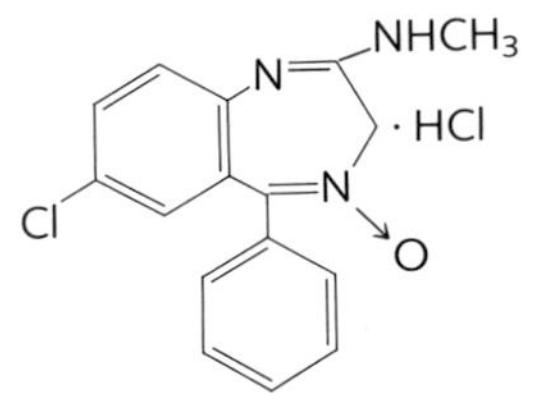

Chlordiazepoxide
hydrochloride
(Librium)

Diazepam
(Valium)

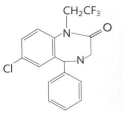

Halazepam
(Paxipam)

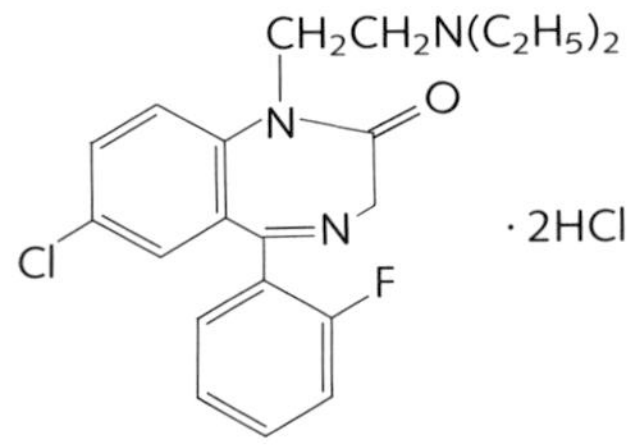

Flurazepam hydrochloride
(Dalmane)

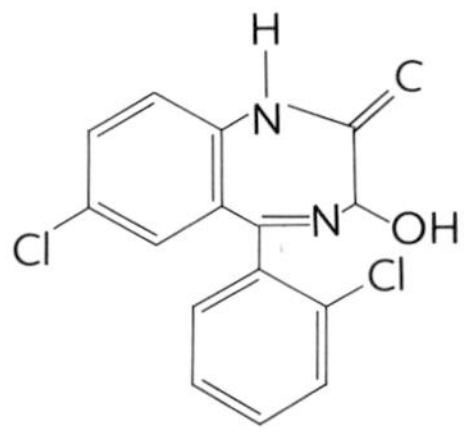

Lorazepam
(Ativan)

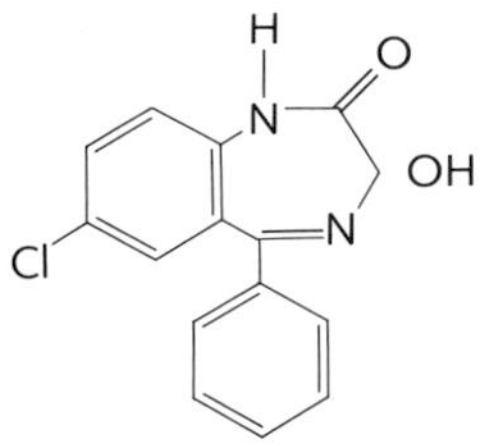

Oxazepam
(Serax)

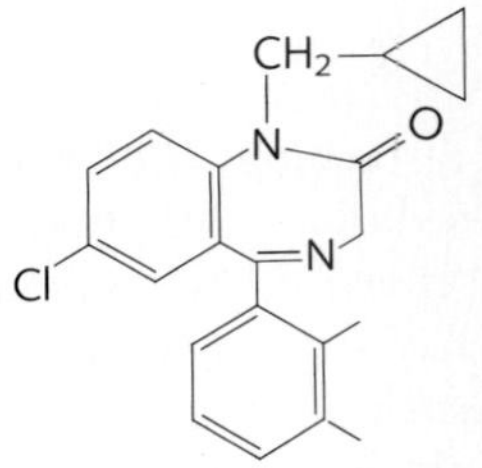

Prazepam
(Centrex)

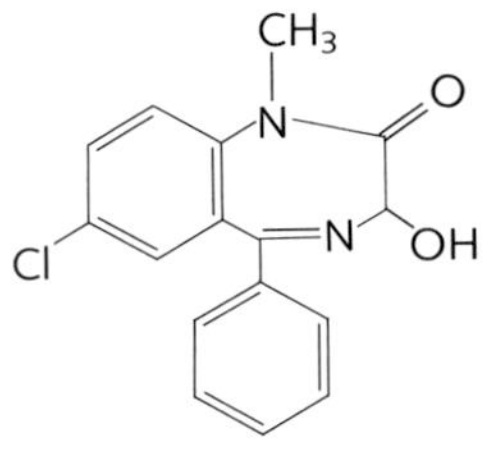

Temazepam
(Restoril)

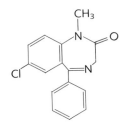

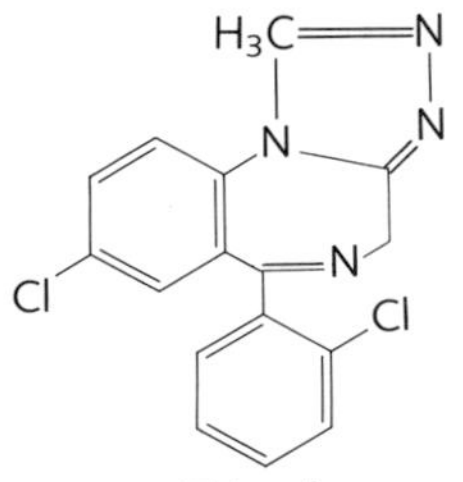

Triazolam
(Halcion)

Chemical structures of important benzodiazepines, barbiturates, convulsants and
drugs that affect the GABA receptor.

Barbiturates

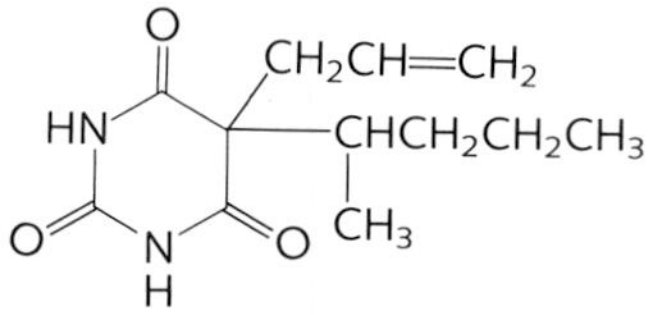

Secobarbital
(Seconal)

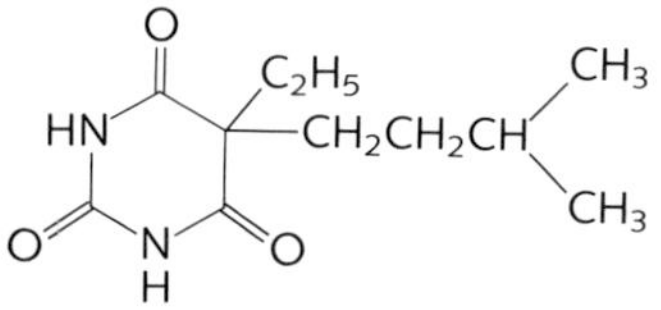

Amobarbital
(Amytal)

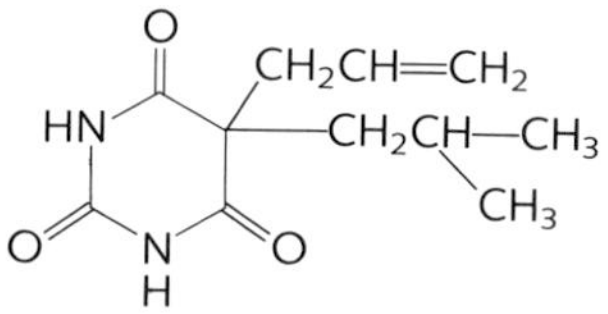

Butalbital

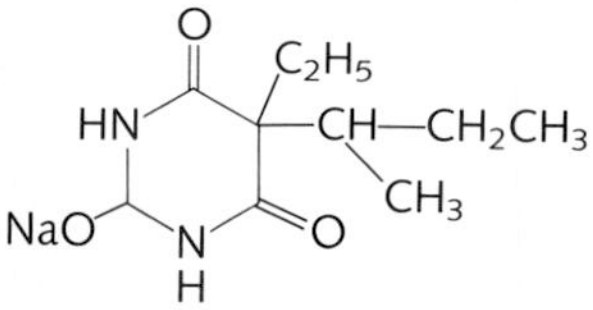

Butabarbital sodium
(Butisol)

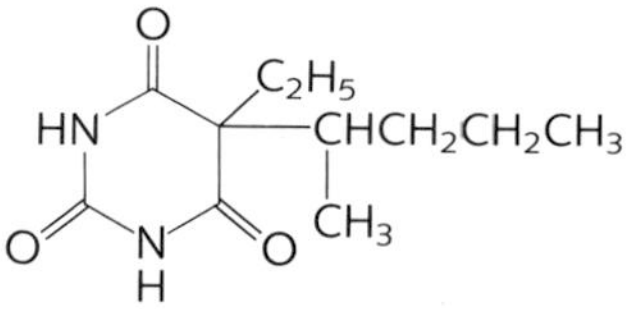

Pentobarbital
(Nembutal)

Mephobarbital
(Mebaral)

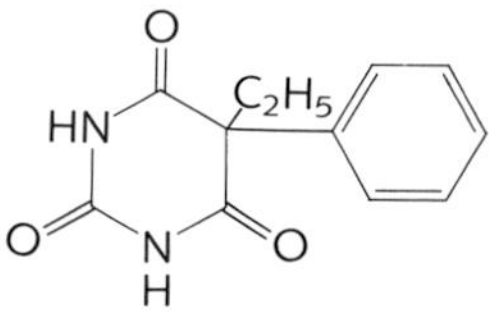

Phenobarbital
(e.g., Luminal)

Convulsants

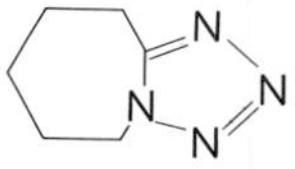

Pentylenetetrazol
(Metrazol)

Picrotoxin

GABA antagonist

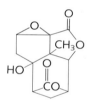

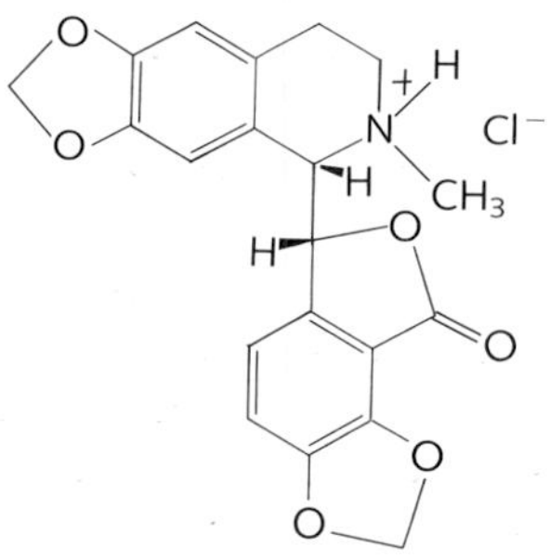

Bicuculline
hydrochloride

Inhibitor of GABA metabolism

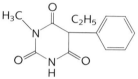

Amino-oxyacetic acid

GABA-mimicking drug

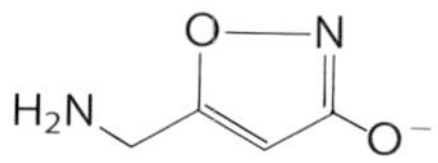

Muscimol

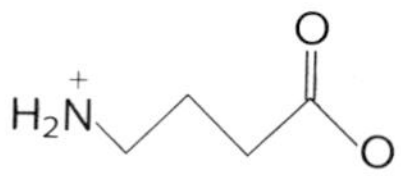

GABA

Ralph Nader's health-research group maintained that excessive use of benzodiazepines in the mid-1970s had created one and a half million American Valium addicts. Senator Edward Kennedy held widely publicized Senate hearings to investigate the situation. Thanks to these and other admonitions, the number of Valium prescriptions filled in 1980 was only half the number filled in the peak year of 1975. Today, the use of benzodiazepines is generally restricted to relatively short-term treatment of anxiety, an application in which the drugs' therapeutic effects will be most evident and their dangers least likely. Patients are given benzodiazepines for a few weeks at the most, during the height of an anxiety attack, and are therefore less likely to become tolerant to and physically dependent upon the drugs.

How Benzodiazepines Act

The apparently selective way in which benzodiazepines relieve anxiety attracted the interest of brain researchers from the start. By studying the molecular mechanisms responsible for those effects, they hoped to gain insight into how the brain normally regulates the emotions that, gone astray, result in feelings of uncontrollable anxiety. The work of the early 1960s established that benzodiazepines, meprobamate, and barbiturates all affect some aspect of synaptic transmission. This was not particularly informative since virtually all psychoactive drugs influence synaptic transmission, but at the time it contributed to the impression that although benzodiazepines were safer and more selective than meprobamate and the barbiturates, all three drug groups had similar pharmacological effects, including sedation and muscle relaxation. Scientists wondered whether this was an indication that the drugs acted at the same or similar recognition sites.

One way of ascertaining whether two drugs act at the same or closely related sites is to make use of the phenomenon of tolerance, one of the components of addiction we discussed in Chapter 2. Barbiturates, meprobamate, and benzodiazepines all induce tolerance. They also display a special relationship know as cross-tolerance, and it is the presence of this effect that suggests they act at similar sites. Cross-tolerance between two drugs means that a person who becomes tolerant to one drug will also prove tolerant to the other, even if the second drug has not been encountered previously (see the illustration on the facing page). Thus, a person treated chronically with a barbiturate will eventually develop a tolerance for it and require substantially larger doses to produce the same behavioral effects. That person would then require a larger dose of meprobamate or of a benzodiazepine than would be necessary if he or she had never become tolerant to the barbiturate. A person treated chronically with benzodiazepines will become cross-tolerant to barbiturates and meprobamate, and a person who is tolerant to meprobamate would be cross-tolerant to benzodiazepines and barbiturates.

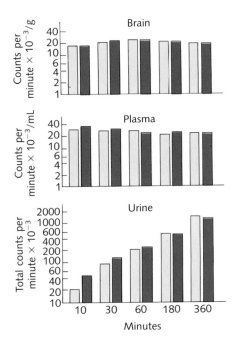

The effects of barbital on normal rats were compared with the effects on rats who had been pretreated with barbital for thirteen days in order to make them tolerant to the drug. In the experiment, tolerant rats and normal controls were each injected with 150 milligrams per kilogram of radioactive barbital. Brain, urine, and blood samples showed that all the rats had roughly the same levels of barbital in their systems. The control rats showed the typical behavioral effects associated with sedatives, all falling asleep by 180 minutes after drug administration. In contrast, the tolerant rats all remained conscious and alert.

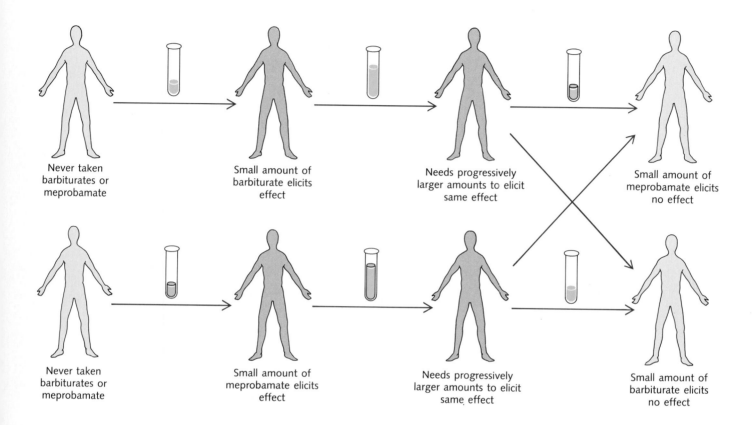

Never taken barbiturates or meprobamate

Small amount of barbiturate elicits effect

Needs progressively larger amounts to elicit same effect

Small amount of meprobamate elicits no effect

Never taken barbiturates or meprobamate

Small amount of meprobamate elicits effect

Needs progressively larger amounts to elicit same effect

Small amount of barbiturate elicits no effect

Cross-dependence between two drugs is analogous to cross-tolerance. It implies that withdrawal symptoms following abrupt termination of one class of drugs can be relieved by treatment with drugs from the other class. Cross-dependence between drugs is put to clinical use in hospitals every day. Barbiturate addicts experiencing withdrawal symptoms are usually treated with benzodiazepines, because the latter are generally considered safer drugs. Delirium tremens, the withdrawal symptoms of alcoholism, are also routinely treated with benzodiazepines.

Cross-tolerance and cross-dependence occur between barbiturates, benzodiazepines, meprobamate, and alcohol. It thus appears that all of the major sedating drugs share similar sites of action. A closer look at the effects of these drugs suggest that barbiturates, meprobamate, and alcohol all act at the same recognition site, while the benzodiazepines act at a different, though related, recognition site. Barbiturates, meprobamate, and alcohol all put animals to sleep at doses only modestly higher than the amounts that produce antianxiety-like behavioral effects. In contrast, benzodiazepines appear to reduce anxiety in animals at doses far lower than those required to put the animals to

Cross-tolerance between barbiturates and meprobamate.

Alcohol

165

sleep. In a number of other behavioral tests, too numerous and complex to review here, the profile of effects at various doses is extremely similar for alcohol, barbiturates, and meprobamate, but measurably different for benzodiazepines. All these results in animals correspond to clinical studies in humans in which benzodiazepines were seen to relieve anxiety at doses that produced minimal sedation, while anxiety-relieving doses of barbiturates, meprobamate, and alcohol were generally unquestionably sedating.

Once they had established that benzodiazepines, barbiturates, and meprobamate all affect synaptic transmission, scientists began to explore the interactions of these drugs with particular neurotransmitters. Some of the most successful research dealt with the neurotransmitter gamma-aminobutyric acid, better known as GABA. GABA is an inhibitory neurotransmitter. When it binds to its receptor sites on neurons, it slows the neuron's rate of firing. Research in the early 1960s showed that these inhibitory effects of GABA were potentiated by alcohol, barbiturates, meprobamate, and benzodiazepines. In these experiments, GABA applied to the surface of neurons in the brain or spinal cord of a cat caused the neuronal firing rate to slow. In cats that had been treated with alcohol, barbiturates, meprobamate, or benzodiazepines, the same amount of slowing was produced by measurably lower doses of GABA.

Although this line of research was promising, it was difficult to follow up in much detail. Obtaining electrical recordings from neurons in the spinal cord of

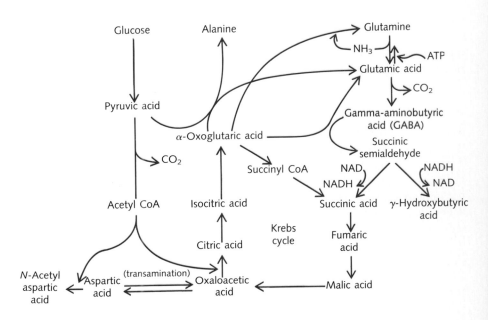

Steps in the metabolism of GABA, and its role in carbohydrate metabolism.

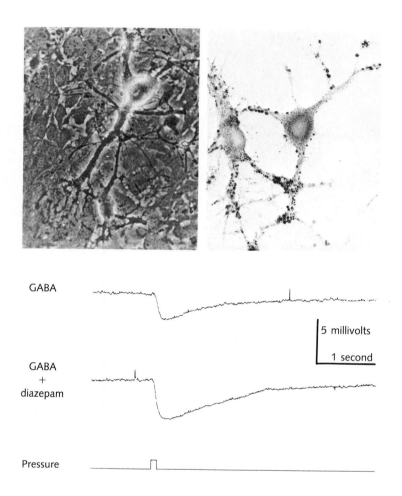

GABA

GABA
+
diazepam

Pressure

5 millivolts

1 second

Electrical tracings compare the response of a mouse spinal cord neuron to GABA alone and in the presence of diazepam. Diazepam appears to increase the effect of GABA, which is an inhibiting neurotransmitter that decreases the nerve membrane's excitability. The photographs show mouse spinal neurons in culture. Dark spots in the photo on the right are made by a stain sensitive to an enzyme at GABA synaptic terminals.

cats was a cumbersome undertaking, and a week of experimentation was required in order to make a thorough characterization of the effect of a single drug. Moreover, these experiments did not demonstrate conclusively that the observed effects on neuronal firing were indeed responsible for the therapeutic actions of the drugs.

A breakthrough occurred in 1977, when two independent groups of researchers discovered the existence of specific benzodiazepine receptors in the brain. Like the discovery of opiate receptors, described in Chapter 2, the identification of benzodiazepine receptors provided a means of understanding what Librium and Valium do at a molecular level, an important advance toward working out how their presence relieves anxiety. Hans Mohler headed one of these groups, under the auspices of the Roche Drug Company in Basel, Switzerland; the other team, Claus Braestrup and Richard Squires, worked at

The first mapping of benzodiazepine receptors in the human brain. *A* Conventional staining, showing different cell groups. *B* Benzodiazepine receptors visible. This image was obtained by adding a radioactive benzodiazepine to a slice of brain tissue. After drug molecules had bound to receptors, the slice was exposed to a photographic emulsion. Radioactive emissions from the drug caused silver grains in the emulsion to develop an image of benzodiazepine-receptor distribution.

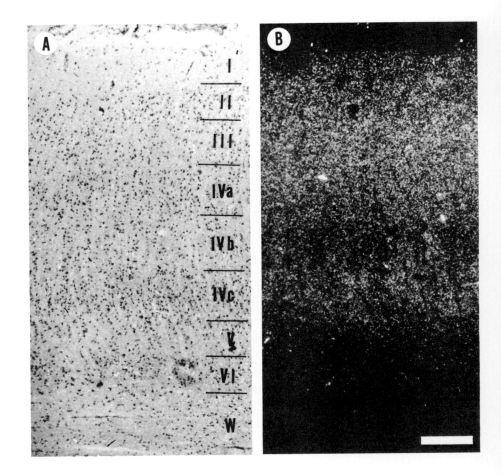

Ferrosan, a small drug company in Denmark. Both teams of researchers were impressed by the way benzodiazepines resembled opiates in terms of their very high potency and extreme selectivity of action. These observations led them to use experimental techniques similar to those that had successfully identified opiate receptors (see Chapter 2). In this case, radioactive Valium was mixed with brain membranes, and it bound to them quite firmly and selectively. To determine whether these binding sites had anything to do with the drugs' behavioral effects, both teams of researchers examined a large number of benzodiazepines. They assessed the potencies of various benzodiazepine drugs in binding to the Valium receptors of brain membranes by determining what concentration of each drug was required to compete with radioactive Valium. If the drug effects were a result of the drugs' actions at receptor sites, a very

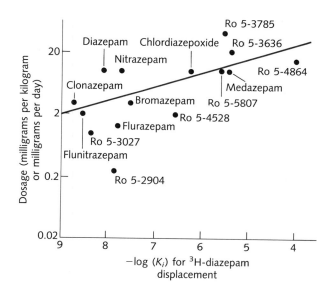

Drug affinities for benzodiazepine receptors correlate with the drugs' potencies as antianxiety agents.

potent benzodiazepine could be present in small amounts and still affect the amount of radioactive Valium that bound to brain membranes. A weaker benzodiazepine would have to be present in higher concentrations in order to compete for the limited number of binding sites. Both groups of investigators found that the relative strengths with which different benzodiazepines bound to the membranes closely paralleled the drugs' antianxiety potencies in humans. The two teams concluded that they had identified the specific sites of benzodiazepine action.

Shortly after the completion of these experiments, benzodiazepine researchers began to ask their version of the question that has proved crucial for understanding the effects of so many psychoactive drugs: "People are not born with Valium in them. What are benzodiazepine receptors doing in the brain?" Did the benzodiazepine receptors normally recognize and bind some already-known neurotransmitter, or did the brain contain a Valium-like neurotransmitter (analogous to the opiatelike enkephalin neurotransmitters) that scientists had yet to discover?

In initial studies, scientists screened numerous neurotransmitters and failed to find any that seemed to bind to benzodiazepine-receptor binding sites. To date, the identification of such a transmitter remains an unresolved controversy, but progress of a sort in this direction (and a remarkable discovery in its own right) was achieved by John Tallman, working at the National Institutes of Mental Health in Bethesda, Maryland, in 1978. Tallman took the same basic approach but examined a wider range of drug concentrations very carefully. Although he did not find a transmitter that bound at the benzodiazepine

Left The effect of varying concentrations of GABAergic drugs on ³H-diazepam binding. *Right* Enhancement of GABA binding by diazepam.

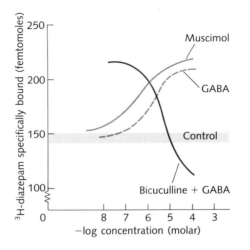

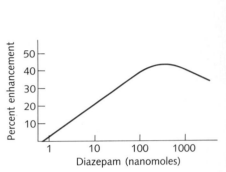

sites, he did learn that the neurotransmitter GABA had a striking effect on those sites. Instead of competing for the same receptor, and thus lowering the amount of radioactive Valium bound to the membranes, GABA *stimulated* the binding of the drug to benzodiazepine-recognition sites (see the chart above). Other researchers then examined GABA receptors directly and found that Valium stimulated the binding of GABA to GABA receptors. The fact that each bound more potently in the other's presence indicated that instead of binding to the identical site, GABA and Valium bind to closely related sites that influence each other. If the benzodiazepine and GABA were competing with each other for the same sites, we would expect GABA to reduce the amount of radioactive Valium binding to the membranes. The only way to explain how GABA enhances the binding of Valium is to assume that, by acting at other, closely related sites, GABA changes the shape of the benzodiazepine receptors so that they can bind Valium more efficiently, thus enabling more radioactive Valium to bind to the receptors.

In these initial experiments, it was not clear where the GABA and benzodiazepine recognition sites were located in relation to each other. Subsequent research has shown that they are actually located on the same large protein molecule. Benzodiazepines stimulate the GABA receptors, facilitating the synaptic actions of GABA, which, you will recall, is an inhibitory neurotransmitter. The calming actions of benzodiazepines are therefore explained by the fact that the drugs enhance GABA's inhibitory effects on neurons in various parts of the brain.

Identifying the parts of the brain in which benzodiazepine receptors are concentrated has added another dimension to our understanding of how the

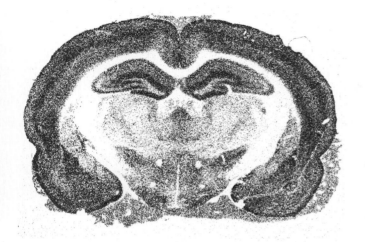 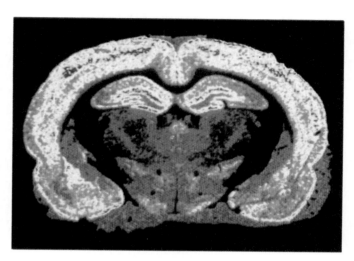

benzodiazepine drugs work. It comes as no surprise that these receptors are most highly concentrated in parts of the brain that regulate emotional behavior, specifically, in the constellation of brain structures known as the limbic system (see the illustration on page 172). Within the limbic system, particularly high concentrations of benzodiazepine receptors are found in the amygdala. This accords well with earlier studies in cats in which manipulations of the amygdala were seen to produce a calming effect on the animals' behavior. The antianxiety effects of benzodiazepines are therefore thought to be mediated through receptors concentrated in limbic structures such as the amygdala. Substantial concentrations of benzodiazepine receptors also occur throughout the cerebral cortex. It is possible that the binding of benzodiazepines to these receptors is responsible for the sedative actions of the drugs.

It seems likely that the benzodiazepine receptor sites are part of a natural mechanism that normally regulates the kinds of emotional states which become altered in patients experiencing symptoms of anxiety. The notion that specific brain systems exist for the purpose of regulating anxietylike states is supported by the actions of some recently developed drugs known as carbolines. These agents bind to the benzodiazepine receptors in the brain, but instead of producing calming effects, the carbolines produce intense anxiety. In the very limited studies in humans that have thus far been conducted, normal volunteers experienced overwhelming anxiety and panic following administration of carboline drugs. This carboline-induced anxiety is far more severe than any emotion that research psychiatrists have observed in neurotically anxious patients, even when patients are in the grip of a panic attack. Since stimulating the receptor (with carbolines) provokes anxiety and modulating the receptor (with benzodiazepines) relieves anxiety, the benzodiazepine

Left Distribution of benzodiazepine receptors in rat forebrain. *Right* Color-coded map of benzodiazepine-receptor distribution in rat brain.

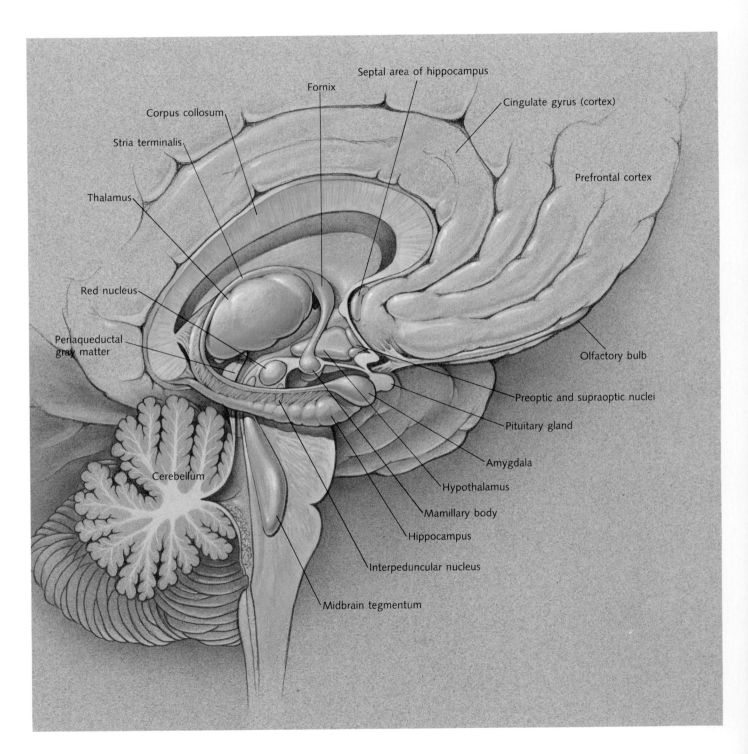

Septal area of hippocampus

Fornix

Corpus collosum

Cingulate gyrus (cortex)

Stria terminalis

Prefrontal cortex

Thalamus

Red nucleus

Periaqueductal
gray matter

Olfactory bulb

Preoptic and supraoptic nuclei

Pituitary gland

Amygdala

Cerebellum

Hypothalamus

Mamillary body

Hippocampus

Interpeduncular nucleus

Midbrain tegmentum

CL 218,872
3-methyl-6-[3-(trifluoromethyl)phenyl]-
1,2,4-triazolo [4,3-b] pyridazine

Zopiclone

Suriclone

receptor would seem to play a role in creating normal and abnormal anxiety.

The ability to evaluate the actions of benzodiazepines at a molecular level and to link these effects to a particular neurotransmitter has greatly accelerated pharmacological research. It is now possible to use benzodiazepine receptors to screen new nonbenzodiazepine drugs that might act at benzodiazepine receptors to affect the emotions in different ways. Numerous nonbenzodiazepine antianxiety drug candidates have been detected with this efficient and economical technique. Many of them could not have been identified by the more conventional tests in intact laboratory animals, which, in any case, permit no more than one or two drugs to be evaluated per week. When benzodiazepine receptors are used to screen new drugs, the pharmacologist can evaluate the therapeutic potential of a different chemical structure in virtually every test tube, assessing a hundred new drug candidates of widely varying structures in a single day. Moreover, conventional techniques require that each substance be tested in a large number of intact animals, necessitating the preparation of at least ten thousand times as much drug as do the new receptor-binding assays. In the past, these and other logistic complications of drug testing made pharmacologists reluctant to test novel chemical structures that had no obvious relationship to the benzodiazepines. Such structures had to be regarded as long shots, unlikely to produce advantageous results. Now that pharmacologists can screen a hundred new chemicals a day for activity at benzodiazepine receptors, there should be much more willingness to evaluate long-shot antianxiety drug candidates.

The Sedative-Convulsant Binding Site

Soon after benzodiazepine receptors had been identified, researchers succeeded in elucidating part of the mechanism through which alcohol, meprobamate, and barbiturates exert their effects. It had been proposed that these sedatives all act at the same site, but this could not be proven by means of direct receptor-binding techniques because the drugs in question are too weak for that

Recently developed nonbenzodiazepine drugs that can act at benzodiazepine receptors. Their clinical effects are essentially the same as those of benzodiazepines. CL 218,872 was the first of the new substances to be discovered.

Facing page Distribution of benzodiazepine receptors in the human brain.

173

method of investigation. The effects of sedatives upon behavior occur only at rather high brain concentrations, while the techniques that had located opiate and benzodiazepine receptors are only applicable with extremely potent drugs that exert their pharmacological actions at very low brain concentrations.

Luckily, previous studies had revealed a selective antagonism between the sedatives and the convulsants. The sedative drugs very potently block the ability of convulsant drugs to produce seizures, and researchers were able to take advantage of that fact. It suggested that the sites affected by sedativelike drugs were related to the sites affected by convulsants. Scientists were also aware that barbiturates are highly effective anticonvulsants (phenobarbital, for example, is widely used to control epilepsy). They therefore tagged potent convulsants with radioactive labels and monitored the convulsants' receptor-binding abilities in the presence of various sedatives. Barbiturates, meprobamate, and alcohol, but not benzodiazepines, appeared to compete directly with convulsants at their binding sites, which are now generally referred to as sedative-convulsant receptors.

As mentioned earlier, similarities in the drugs' actions suggested to scientists that the sedative-binding site was closely related to the benzodiazepine-binding site. This was supported by the finding that barbiturates, alcohol, and meprobamate function like benzodiazepines in facilitating the synaptic effects of GABA. Given the various lines of evidence, researchers now had a fairly clear idea of how antianxiety and sedative drugs might act. They theorized that the sedative-convulsant, GABA, and benzodiazepine receptors lay close to each other in a large receptor complex, perhaps a single large protein responsible for the actions of all of these drugs. GABA and the benzodiazepines acted on one subdivision of the protein (what protein chemists call a subunit), though they did not bind to the same site, and sedatives and convulsants acted on a different subdivision (these two types of drugs did compete for the same site). The binding of drugs to one subunit altered the way that drugs interacted with the other subunit.

The next breakthrough in explaining the clinical effects of benzodiazepines and sedatives represented valuable progress in elucidating the process of synaptic transmission in general. Specifically, scientists have now learned how one neurotransmitter, GABA, is able to alter, in this case inhibit, the rate of neuronal firing. Neurophysiologists had established that GABA exerts its inhibitory effects by widening the chloride-ion channels in the neuronal membrane. When GABA binds to its receptors, the chloride channels enlarge, and chloride ions are freer to move from the outside to the inside of the nerve cell. This changes the internal electrical charge of the cell in such a way that the cell is less likely to fire. However, nobody knew just how the GABA receptor was linked to the chloride-ion channel, or, indeed, how *any* neurotransmitter receptor was linked to any ion channel. Were the neurotransmitter receptors and the ion channels located close to each other in the nerve membrane, or were they far apart? How many molecules composed each system? Might they even

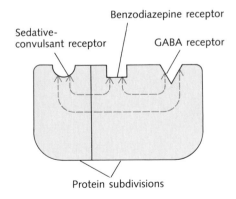

Sedative-convulsant receptor | Benzodiazepine receptor | GABA receptor

Protein subdivisions

A single protein molecule contains binding sites for GABA, benzodiazepines, and sedatives and convulsants.

be part of the same molecule? Such matters are fundamental to understanding synaptic transmission, which in turn is one of the most fundamental processes in the brain.

When scientists began to test the effects of various ions on the GABA-benzodiazepine-sedative-convulsant receptor complex, the answer became evident. Researchers found that unless they added a good amount of chloride to the test tube, they could not detect the slightest interaction of barbiturate or convulsant molecules with their receptors. This suggested that the sedative-convulsant receptor was in fact a portion of the chloride-ion channel, and that a drug's sedating or convulsant actions reflected the compound's effect on the passage of chloride ions into the post-synaptic neuron. By adding chloride ions to the test tube, researchers had learned they could detect something as complicated as a channel in a membrane that opens and closes in response to neurotransmitters.

The initial studies on chloride and receptors employed brain membranes. Very recently, however, Eric Barnard, at Imperial College in London, managed to separate the GABA-benzodiazepine-sedative-convulsant receptor complexes from the rest of the brain-membrane components and, after several years of careful purification, to isolate a single protein molecule. In this one protein he was able to detect the binding sites for GABA, benzodiazepines, and barbiturates and convulsants. Moreover, the isolated receptor protein displayed sensitivity to chloride ions. This was final proof that a single protein molecule contains the recognition sited for the neurotransmitter GABA and for all the various drugs that influence GABA neurotransmission. As expected, the protein is made up of several subunits, one of which appears to possess separate binding sites for GABA and benzodiazepines. These sites are apparently located close to each other and constructed in such a way that the binding of GABA increases the binding of benzodiazepines (see the diagrams opposite and on page 176). As researchers had expected, a distinct subunit of the protein has a site for both sedative drugs—such as alcohol, barbiturates, and meprobamate—and convulsant drugs. The sedative-convulsant receptor and the GABA and benzodiazepine receptors can interact with one another, explaining why sedatives such as barbiturates can change the binding of radioactive Valium to benzodiazepine receptors. Similarly, benzodiazepines alter the binding of radioactive convulsants to the sedative-convulsant receptors. These close interactions may account for the striking synergistic interactions between benzodiazepines and alcohol or barbiturates in which relatively low doses of Valium can prove lethal to someone under the influence of alcohol or barbiturates. Unfortunately, it is still not at all clear why the binding of a benzodiazepine to its receptor produces a selective antianxiety effect while the binding of a sedative to its closely related receptor mediates a sedating effect.

The most remarkable characteristic of the protein isolated by Barnard is that it also contains the chloride-ion channel. Thus, when a molecule of GABA binds to its receptor, it affects the size of a chloride-ion channel that is located

Relation of the GABA-benzodiazepine-sedative-convulsant receptor to the chloride channel. *A,B* Increased levels of GABA enhance the entrance of chloride ions into the nerve cell. *C* Benzodiazepine enhances the effect of GABA, so that basal levels of GABA enlarge the chloride ion channel. *D* Benzodiazepine antagonists prevent enhancement of GABA effects but do not reduce basal chloride ion conductance. *E* GABA antagonists prevent enlargement of chloride channels in spite of presence of benzodiazepines. *F* Presence of valproate, a sedative, results in a widening of the chloride ion channel in the presence of basal levels of GABA. *G* Presence of picrotoxin, a convulsant, prevents widening of chloride ion channel, even in the presence of large amounts of GABA.

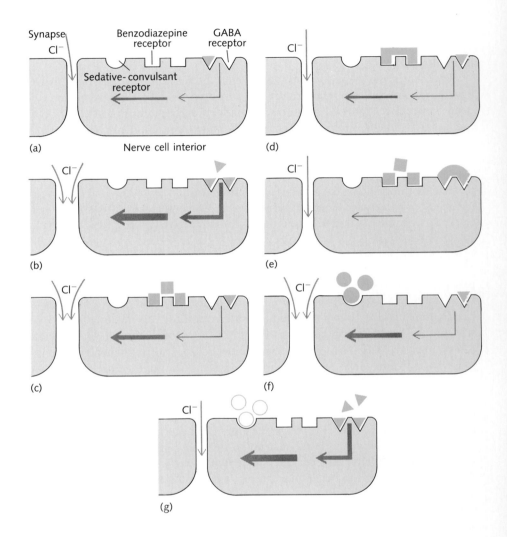

near it in the same large protein. Now scientists can explore how the recognition of GABA at its receptor site changes the protein's three-dimensional structure so as to enlarge the chloride-ion channel. Indeed, one can ask just what a chloride-ion channel looks like in a protein molecule. Presumably, the ion channel is circular in cross section and extends like a cylinder through the neuronal membrane. Are the chains of amino acids wrapped about in a circular fashion, so that a head-on view of the channel would resemble a donut? Do the convulsant drugs themselves fit into the hole of the donut, or do they bind to nearby sites on the protein? How far apart on the receptor protein are the sites where GABA and benzodiazepines bind? There is much for researchers to accomplish in coming years, but the rapid escalation of new insights suggests that some of the remaining questions will soon be answered. We can anticipate great progress, both in our fundamental understanding of brain function and in our ability to develop newer, more effective, and safer drugs with which to treat anxiety.

Up until this point in the book, most of what we have learned about brain mechanisms has revolved around the ways in which psychoactive drugs alter the feelings that clothe our perceptions of the world around us. The next chapter represents something of a departure from this pattern. In it we will examine a group of substances that seem to undermine our most basic, and generally most dependable, sensory perceptions, and we will discuss what these drugs have begun to tell us about how we sense the dimensions of space and time and our own integrity within them.

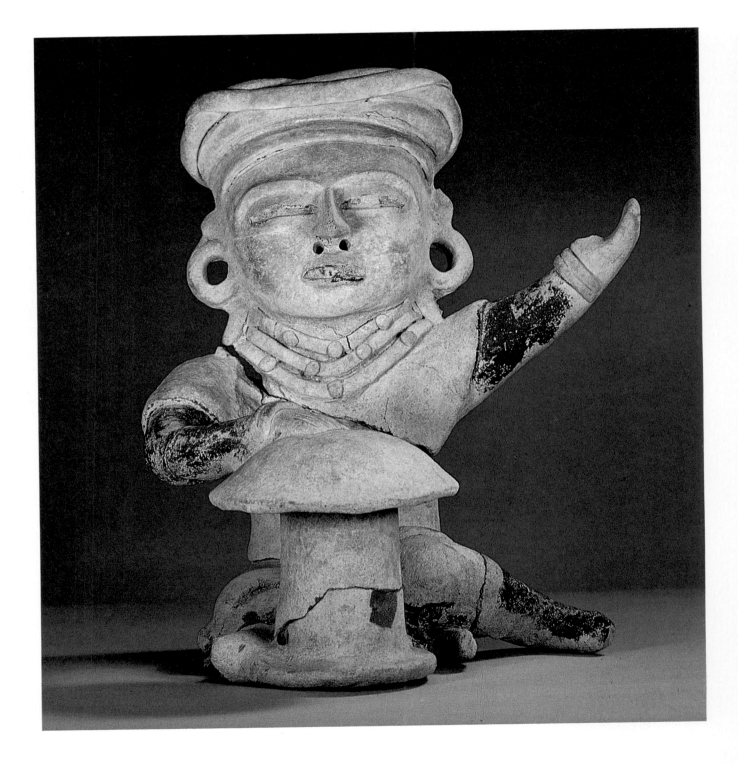

Enlightenment in a Pill

From the pharmacologist's point of view, psychedelic drugs are agents of negligible worth. A person whose vocation is to develop drugs that relieve symptoms and, if possible, cure diseases has little use for a class of compounds with no demonstrated therapeutic use, a history of extensive abuse, and the ability to provoke psychosis. Yet many brain researchers value the psychedelic agents above any of the other psychoactive drugs. These scientists are immensely interested in understanding why the changes wrought by LSD, mescaline, and psilocybin seem to affect the very core of the user's consciousness. They want to know the molecular mechanisms that underlie the psychedelic experience, hoping thereby to discover the physiological principles behind such intangible yet ineluctable entities as our sense of religiousness, our striving for immortality, and our fundamental awareness of being human. To put it more prosaically, by studying the actions of psychedelic drugs, scientists hope to learn about the brain processes responsible for the way that we perceive both ourselves and our relationship with the world outside ourselves.

The Psychedelic Experience

Experienced drug users talk about subtle distinctions between the effects of the various psychedelic substances. For instance, mescaline is said to provide a more sensual, visual experience while LSD has a stronger effect on one's sense of self. LSD is the best known of the psychedelic drugs, but a wide range of chemical agents—mescaline, psilocybin, and a series of compounds whose names read like an alphabet soup of bureaucratic designations (DOM, DOET, MDA, MDMA, and many more)—all produce the same basic effects.

The first change one is likely to notice after taking a psychedelic drug are changes in sensory perception, especially visual perception. I recall this from my own experimentation with LSD, which took place in a Victorian house on

Facing page Terra-cotta figurine from the Remojadas culture near Veracruz, Mexico, depicts a female shaman and a magic mushroom.

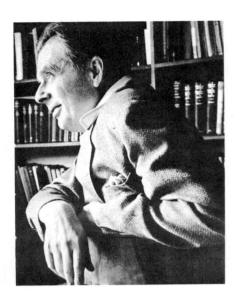

English writer Aldous Huxley (1894–1963), whose 1954 essay *The Doors of Perception* describes an encounter with mescaline.

one of the slopes of Twin Peaks, the highest hill in San Francisco. At first, the only notable difference was the appearance of a slight purplish fringe around the objects in my vicinity. Next, every object I focused on began to seem amusingly quaint. The rooftops and facades of houses reminded me of the gingerbread house in "Hansel and Gretel," which observation caused me to giggle uncontrollably. As I became more and more entranced by these and other visual sensations, the giggly feeling gradually changed to awe. I looked at the faces of the people around me and noticed details of their physiognomy that had never struck me before. Each pore in my companions' skin was now visible, and every facial expression was laden with significance. As I looked on each person's face I empathized with the exact emotion I thought I saw expressed. At that point, the distortions became more extreme. If I focused upon my forefinger, it would swell. If I concluded that the finger was unimportant, it literally shrank into insignificance. When I gazed at the intricate woodwork that edged the ceiling, the carved designs would undulate back and forth.

My experiences were by no means unique. Countless others have noticed similar perceptual changes under the influence of psychedelic drugs. *The Doors of Perception* is British writer Aldous Huxley's eloquent description of twelve hours under the influence of a single capsule of mescaline. "Half an hour after swallowing the drug I became aware of a slow dance of golden lights. A little later there were sumptuous red surfaces swelling and expanding from bright nodes of energy that vibrated with a continuously changing, patterned light." Like many others who have used psychedelic drugs, Huxley was especially taken with the images he saw when he closed his eyes: "At another time, the closing of my eyes revealed a complex of grey structures, within which pale blueish spheres kept emerging into intense solidity and, having emerged, would slide noiselessly upwards, out of sight."

One of the most incredible perceptual changes wrought by psychedelic drugs is referred to as synesthesia. This is a phenomenon in which the senses become transmuted, so that touch may be experienced as sound, sound as vision, and so forth. In my own case, about an hour after ingesting the LSD, I clapped my hands and saw sound waves passing before my eyes. When two people clapped their hands at different sound frequencies, I saw two sets of waves that differed in magnitude and seemed to collide with each other. No one had ever told me about synesthesia, and I did not read about it until months later, so it was not an experience I had been conditioned to expect. However, I wonder whether I would have "seen" the sound waves if high school physics had not taught me that they exist.

Vision and hearing are not the only senses affected by the drugs. The sense of time is likewise markedly distorted. Two hours after taking the drug, I felt I had been under its influence for thousands of years. The remainder of my life on the planet Earth seemed to stretch ahead into infinity, and at the same time I felt infinitely old. When I tried to play the guitar, every quarter note seemed to linger for a month. Aldous Huxley describes having a similar experience while gazing at the legs of a chair: "How miraculous their tubularity, how supernatural their polished smoothness! I spent several minutes—or was it several centuries?—not merely gazing at those bamboo legs, but actually *being* them."

The sense of space is altered, too. I remember walking from one room to the next with a feeling of having crossed the breadth of the universe. I climbed the stairs to the second floor and looked back down on events that were surely taking place 400,000 miles away.

As riotous as these changes can be, even more extraordinary is the ineffable change that takes place in the user's sense of self. Boundaries between self and nonself evaporate, giving rise to a serene sense of being at one with the universe. I recall muttering to myself again and again, "All is one, all is one." My wife, who was the sober "observer" for the day, became alarmed and asked me what was going on, to which I could only reply, "What matters? All is one."

This transcending of ego boundaries is experienced by almost everyone who takes a psychedelic drug. Aldous Huxley commented, "To others again is revealed the glory, the infinite value and meaningfulness of naked existence, of the given, unconceptualized event. In the final stage of egolessness there is an obscure knowledge that All is in awe—that Awe is actually each. This is as near, I take it, as a finite mind can ever come to perceiving everything that is happening everywhere in the universe."

Of course, dissolution of the ego, loss of one's sense of self, has its dangers as well as its attractions. A loss of ego boundaries is one of the hallmarks of psychotic disintegration, according to psychiatric dogma. In my own case, the powerful feeling of oneness with the universe was followed by a loss of awareness of just who I was. I began to call out, "Who am I? Where is the world?" At the height of this disintegration, I was terrified. I tried frantically to remember my name—hoping thus to recapture reality—but it eluded me. In the end, I grasped at the one name I could think of: "San Francisco." I repeated it again and again, "San Francisco, San Francisco, San Francisco." It seemed to be a clue to where I was and who I might be. By this time, eight hours after consuming the LSD, the drug's effects began to wear off. By clinging to the notion that San Francisco was a relevant place, I gradually managed to remember who I was, where I was, and the identities of the people there with me. Very quickly, the world about me coalesced, and reality supervened.

Aldous Huxley had a similar experience: "I found myself all at once on the brink of panic. This, I suddenly thought, was going too far. Too far, even though the going was into intenser beauty, deeper significance. The fear, as I analyzed it in retrospect, was of being overwhelmed, of disintegrating under a pressure of reality greater than a mind, accustomed to living most of the time in a cozy world of symbols, could possibly bear."

The panic can be far more devastating than mine was. Terror and confusion have caused many people in these circumstances to jump from windows to their deaths. Others have suffered psychotic breakdowns from which they failed to emerge when the drug's effects wore off. Hundreds of cases of schizophrenic illness have been precipitated by a single psychedelic drug experience. The possibility that they may initiate a long-term mental illness is perhaps the most serious danger presented by psychedelic drugs.

How were pharmacologists to classify such a remarkable group of substances? LSD and its relatives were first referred to as hallucinogens, but that characterization was soon abandoned because the drugs do not produce frank hallucinations. A hallucination is a perception that takes place in the absence of an environmental stimulus. According to this definition, the psychedelic drug experience is rarely hallucinatory. These drugs do not create perceptions, they cause existing perceptions to be *distorted*. Some pharmacologists designated the drugs psychotomimetic, which translates as "drugs that induce psychotic states." It cannot be denied that one is indeed psychotic under the influence of typical doses employed by most users; however, many other drugs also induce psychoses in adequate doses. We saw in Chapter 5 that overuse of cocaine or amphetamine elicits a paranoid schizophrenia–like state. Drugs such as atropine and scopolamine, which block acetylcholine receptors, are also capable of causing psychotic states. The trait that truly distinguishes the psychedelic drugs from drugs in other classes is the way psychedelic drugs

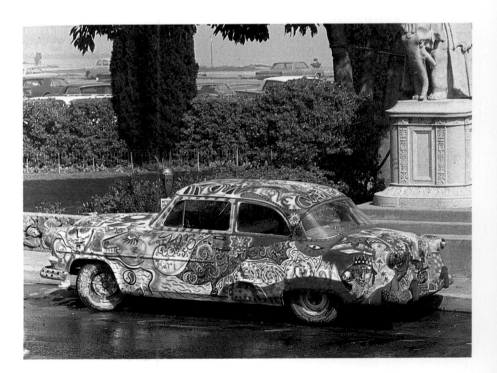

The psychedelic art of the 1960s attempted to convey the kinds of sensations induced by psychedelic drugs.

intensify the perceptual and conceptual aspects of mental function. The term psychedelic was coined by the psychiatrist Humphrey Osmond in an effort to emphasize these features: "I have tried to find an appropriate name for the agents under discussion, a name that will include the concepts of enriching the mind and enlarging the vision. . . . My choice, because it is clear, euphonious, and uncontaminated by other associations, is psychedelic, mind manifesting."

Mental States Mimicked by Psychedelic Drugs

The foregoing description of an LSD experience may sound more like poetry than science, but I felt it was relevant to describe the almost unbelievable changes that take place in normal human beings when they consume psychedelic drugs. The alterations in sensory perception, sense of time and space, and sense of self are so alien to everyday experience that they shed new light on the workings of these everyday mental functions. For instance, the knowledge that psychedelic drugs can elicit synesthesia led brain scientists to search for neuronal mechanisms that might equate different sensory processes such as sight and sound, and the almost predictable transcendence of ego boundaries brought on by these drugs has caused scientists to consider that there might be a neural basis for the ego.

Most of the mind-altering drugs we examined in previous chapters can be characterized by the different ways they impair mental processes and dull the sensibilities. This cannot be said of psychedelic drugs, which, if anything, make people hyperalert, so that every moment of the experience is inscribed indelibly upon their consciousness and remembered vividly. Though the drugs distort perception and cognition, users have a subjective sense that awareness is being heightened and that the changes in seeing, hearing, and thinking may reflect more "reality" than they are attuned to in their normal state of consciousness. Psychedelic drug enthusiasts maintain that the new level of experience revealed by these agents is literally "superhuman" and far closer to the supernatural than anything humans can attain by other means. Students of Christian, Buddhist, and other forms of mysticism have often commented on the similarity of the psychedelic experience to the transcendental state attained through Zen or other forms of deep meditation.

Walter N. Pahnke, a psychiatrist who, before entering medical school, had earned a doctor of divinity degree, conducted a systematic experiment to determine whether a psychedelic drug, psilocybin, could provoke experiences similar to mystical religious experiences. On Good Friday in 1962, twenty theological students, all of whom claimed to have had previous mystical religious experiences, received a drug they were told was psilocybin. Actually, only half received psilocybin. The other half were given nicotinic acid, a B vitamin that causes no perceptional distortions, only a sensation of warmth and a tingling on the skin, which are also minor side effects of psilocybin. Three of the ten students who took psilocybin had profound mystical experiences, very much

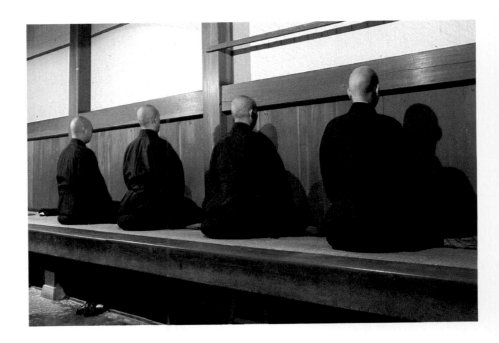

Japanese monks practicing Za-Zen meditation. Advocates of psychedelic drugs say that drugs like LSD and mescaline bring the same transcendence and enlightenment that many people claim to achieve through meditation.

like what they had experienced earlier in a drug-free religious trance. None of those receiving nicotinic acid reported experiencing such effects.

Uses and Actions of Psychedelic Drugs

Mescaline   Like any number of pharmacological agents in use today, psychedelic agents trace their descent from the plant extracts of folk medicine. Because of their remarkable effects upon the mind, these particular agents were likely to be incorporated into the religious practices of the early cultures that discovered them. Peyote, the plant from which mescaline is obtained, has been employed for centuries in the religious ceremonies of Mexican Indians.

Peyote is a cactus designated either as *Lophophora williamsii* or *Anhalonium lewinii*. Much of what we know about its early use comes from Francisco Hernández, court physician to King Philip II of Spain. Hernández made several trips to Mexico, the first together with Cortez, for the purpose of gathering information about Indian herbal medicines. He learned that the Aztecs regarded the peyote cactus as sacred and noted, "Those who eat or chew it see visions either frightful or laughable . . . terrifying sights like the Devil."

Peyote was the key to the religious activities of the Mexican Indians and persists to this day as one of their sacraments. Instead of resisting Christianity, Mexican Indians integrated the two religions, combining the teachings of

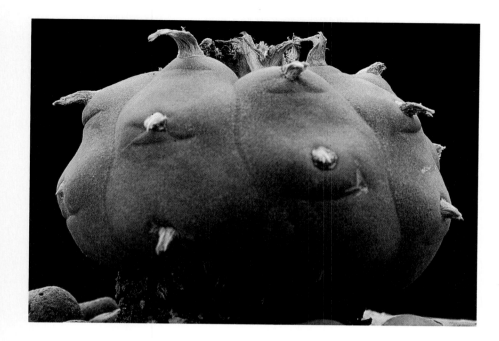

Lophophora williamsii, the peyote cactus.

Christianity with their own traditional religious practices. Gradually the religion of peyotism spread to Indians in territories that now form part of the United States. In 1918, the cult received official sanction as the Native American Church of the United States, formally amalgamating Christianity and traditional Indian beliefs. In the 1960s, it was regarded as the major religious cult of American Indians between the Rocky Mountains and the Mississippi. The use by the Native American Church of a mind-altering drug became the subject of legal and congressional legislative dispute, but at present peyotism is completely legal.

Peyote contains many chemical constituents. A German researcher, A. Heffter, identified mescaline as the plant's major active ingredient in 1896. E. Spaeth, another German chemist, worked out the compound's chemical structure in 1918. As always, the availability of the drug in a pure form facilitated extensive studies of its pharmacological effects. However, aficianados of peyote never fail to remind chemists that ingesting mescaline is not identical to consuming peyote, since other substances in the peyote plant may contribute to the total psychological experience. There may well be subtle differences in the effects of peyote and mescaline, but they are difficult to specify and examine.

Methoxyamphetamines   Mescaline is a relatively weak drug. To experience its psychedelic effects, the user must consume several hundred milligrams, an

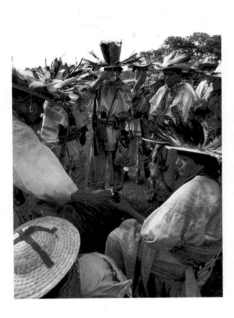

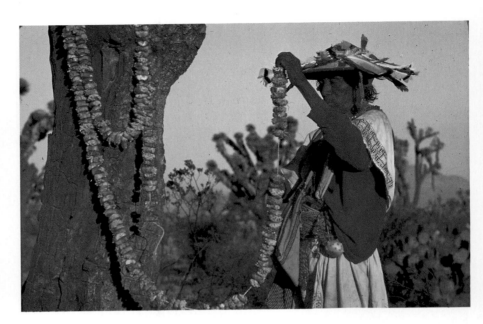

Left A Huichol Indian shaman receiving peyote during a ritual ceremony. *Right* A shaman stringing peyote up for drying.

amount that can cause intestinal upset. Alexander Shulgin, a chemist at the Dow Chemical Company research laboratories outside San Francisco, worked throughout the 1960s to enhance the potency of mescaline by modifying the mescaline molecule. He began by adding a methyl group to the side chain, a change that yielded TMA, the amphetamine derivative of mescaline (see the chemical structures on page 188). This methyl group increases the drug's potency by preventing the enzymatic removal of the side-chain nitrogen, a first step in the metabolism of mescaline. Shulgin then moved the methoxy groups about the ring and converted some of them to other types of groups. These changes, too, augmented the potency of the resulting compound. Low doses of some of the methoxyamphetamines seem to cause enhanced self-awareness without producing psychotic effects or visual distortions. At Johns Hopkins, we showed this to be the case for DOET.

Certain of Shulgin's methoxyamphetamines were subsequently manufactured by illicit laboratories and sold on the streets of San Francisco and other cities. MDMA, popularly designated "ecstasy," has become particularly sought after in the 1980s. It is said to act like DOET, augmenting self-awareness at low doses and eliciting euphoria, the latter perhaps due in part to the drug's amphetamine-like properties. Psychotherapists have used it, in violation of federal law, as an adjunct to insight-oriented therapy. DOM, another compound developed by Shulgin, achieved national notoriety in the late 1960s because of its widespread use in San Francisco's Haight-Ashbury district and the "bad trips" associated with its prolonged effects.

186

Psychedelic drugs

Lysergic acid diethylamide (LSD)	Semisynthetic, extremely potent, acting at a tenth of a milligram dosage.
Mescaline	Active ingredient of peyote cactus, chemically similar to norepinephrine.
Tryptamines	Related in structure to serotonin.
Psilocybin	The active ingredient in certain Mexican mushrooms. In the body, its phosphate group is removed, forming the active product psilocin.
Psilocin	The active metabolite of psilocybin.
Dimethyltryptamine	Totally synthetic. Not active orally, so is injected or inhaled. Shortest duration of action of all psychedelic drugs, about 45 minutes.
Methoxyamphetamines	Totally synthetic; an additional methyl group on the side chain converts mescaline into a methoxyamphetamine. This chemical modification slows metabolism and in some methoxyampetamines confers an amphetamine-like alerting effect along with psychedelic actions.
3,4,5-Trimethoxy-amphetamine (3,4,5-TMA)	The amphetamine derivative directly corresponding to mescaline.
DOM (STP)	Chemically, 2,5-dimethoxy-4-methylamphetamine. About 50 to 100 times more potent than mescaline owing to changes in location of methoxy groups as well as addition of a methyl group. In the late 1960s DOM was extremely popular among San Francisco hippies because of its long duration of action. It was popularly known as STP, so named as an abbreviation for *Serenity, Tranquility, Peace,* and as a play on the name of the gasoline additive.
MDMA (Ecstasy)	Chemically, 3,4-methylenedioxy-*N*-methylamphetamine. Popular in the 1980s because of reports that in low doses it confers euphoria and enhanced self-awareness without producing psychotic effects and visual distortions. Some psychotherapists have used it (illicitly) to help enhance their patients' insight. In rats it appears to damage serotonin neurons.
DOET	Chemically, 2,5-dimethoxy-4-ethylamphetamine, the ethyl derivative of DOM. Experimental studies in normal volunteers at Johns Hopkins demonstrated effects like those claimed for MDMA, namely, enhanced self-awareness at low doses without visual distortions or psychosis.

Chemical structures of methoxyamphetamines.

Mescaline

3,4,5-Trimethoxyamphetamine
(TMA)

2,5-Dimethoxy-4-methylamphetamine
(DOM, STP)

2,5-Dimethoxy-4-ethylamphetamine
(DOET)

3,4-Methylenedioxy-*N*-methylamphetamine
(MDMA, Ecstasy)

The Magic Mushroom   The "magic mushroom" of Mexico and Central America has a longer history of human use than any other mind-altering plant. Stone sculptures of psychoactive mushrooms found in El Salvador, Guatemala, and parts of Mexico date well before 500 B.C. Faces of gods or demons sculpted on the stems emphasize the mushrooms' role in religious ritual, which is also evident from their Indian name, teonanactl, meaning "food of the gods." Priests who accompanied Cortez to Mexico recorded rituals employing teonanactl as well as peyote: "Some saw in a vision that they would die in war. Some saw in a vision that they would be devoured by wild beasts. . . . Some saw in a vision that they would pass to tranquility in death. . . . All such things they saw . . . and when [the effects of] the mushroom ceased, they conversed with one another, and spoke of what they had seen in the vision."

In contrast to the public character of the peyote cult, the properties and rituals of the magic mushroom were engulfed in secrecy. Europeans and Americans knew of the religion's existence and had heard of the psychoactive mushroom, but few if any had witnessed any ceremonial events. Credit for making the first inroads into the teonanactl culture and bringing back large batches of the mushrooms for chemical identification belongs to a remarkable husband and wife team. R. Gordon Wasson was a vice-president of the J.P. Morgan Bank in New York, and his wife, Valentina, was a pediatrician with an interest in the medicinal effects of plants. In the early 1950s, they made several expeditions to Mexico, for the purpose of insinuating themselves into the Indian culture and obtaining the teonanactl plant. Finally, in 1955, they were permitted to join in a sacred mushroom ceremony, to ingest the substances, and to acquire samples. The Wassons were accompanied by a mushroom expert, mycologist Roger Heim, who identified the psychoactive mushroom as a member of the genus *Psilocybe*. The fungus was thereafter designated *Psilocybe mexicana*.

The next task was to identify the active ingredient. After a number of unsuccessful collaborations with chemists in Europe and the United States, Heim enlisted the assistance of Albert Hofmann at the Sandoz Drug Company in Basel, Switzerland. Hofmann was already famous as the discoverer of LSD. In a little less than a year, he succeeded in isolating the active component of *Psilocybe mexicana*.

The first step in isolating the active chemical of a psychoactive plant is to establish a test system to monitor pharmacological activity throughout the

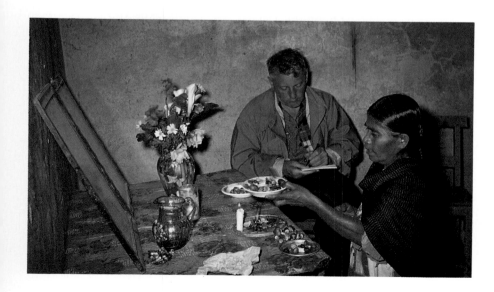

Gordon Wasson (1898–   ) during a 1956 expedition to Mexico, with *curandera* (medicine woman) Maria Sabina.

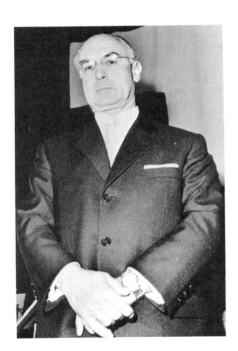

Psilocin

Psilocybin

course of purification. In an attempt to set up such a test system, Hofmann administered mushroom extracts to mice, dogs, and other animals, but he saw no behavioral changes reproducible enough to use as an index of the purification process. Fearing that the mushroom extracts had already lost their biological activity he ingested some of the material himself. The dramatic effects he experienced convinced him that the material was indeed active and virtually indistinguishable from LSD. Thereafter, as Hofmann proceeded with the purification, he tested every successive fraction on himself.

In early 1958, Hofmann isolated psilocybin and psilocin, two pure chemicals that appeared to account for all the psychoactive effects of the mushroom. Soon he and his colleagues at Sandoz had worked out the chemical structures, which are identical except for the presence of a phosphorus atom in the psilocybin molecule. In the body, this phosphorus is almost immediately removed, which means that the mushroom's effects are actually mediated through a single chemical, psilocin. Hofmann and his colleagues were amazed by the close structural similarity between psilocybin, psilocin, and the neurotransmitter serotonin. They were also impressed with the two drugs' clinical resemblance to LSD, the principal difference being that the effects of psilocybin and psilocin wear off after four to six hours, whereas the effects of LSD persist for eight to twelve. Another difference is that, on a weight basis, psilocybin and psilocin are less than 1 percent as active as LSD.

Lysergic Acid Diethylamide   The best known of all the psychedelic drugs is lysergic acid diethylamide, or LSD. It was synthesized by Albert Hofmann fully twenty years before he isolated psilocybin and psilocin. Of course, mescaline had been known previously, but LSD was the first psychedelic agent to have a major impact on Western culture. The altered state of consciousness induced by LSD contributed greatly to the philosophical outlook of American youth in the mid-1960s, giving rise to the "hippy rebellion," the counterculture that began in the Haight-Ashbury district of San Francisco and then spread throughout the United States and Europe.

LSD is a semisynthetic preparation derived from ergot, an extract of the fungus *Claviceps purpurea,* which grows as a parasite on rye wheat. Ergot was first recognized as a poison. In the Middle Ages, frequent mass outbreaks of a toxic condition known as ergotism caused arms or legs to develop dry gangrene that eventually necessitated amputation. Ergotism was also associated with frequently fatal convulsions. Surprisingly, by the late Middle Ages this dreaded fungus was being used for medical purposes. Midwives employed it to contract the uterus and precipitate childbirth. Ergot was a mainstay of nineteenth-century American obstetrics, as well, employed to prevent bleeding after childbirth by inducing a vigorous and prolonged contraction of the uterus.

Organic chemists isolated various chemicals from the ergot plant. The first of these, obtained in pure form by Arthur Stoll at the Sandoz Drug Company

Albert Hofmann (1906–   ), the Swiss chemist who in 1943 discovered LSD.

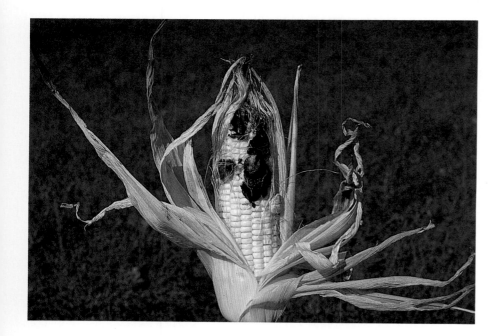

An ear of corn infested with *Claviceps* fungus, the source of ergot.

in 1918, was called ergotamine. Among other effects, ergotamine contracts the superficial blood vessels of the head. To this day, it is the most consistently effective acute treatment for migraine headache. In the 1930s, several Sandoz researchers, including Stoll, isolated the chemical in ergot that causes contractions of the uterus. They called the compound ergonovine. At about the same time, chemists at the Rockefeller Institute in New York identified the common nucleus of all the ergot chemicals and named it lysergic acid.

The various active components of ergot were present in only very small quantities in the ergot fungus. The availability of lysergic acid enabled pharmacologists to synthesize these compounds in larger amounts. Thus, in the mid-1930s Hofmann worked out a synthetic procedure to produce large amounts of ergonovine, which soon became the major drug in obstetrics for precipitating labor and stopping postpartum bleeding. He then clarified the chemical structure of a mixture of ergots earlier designated ergotoxine because of their toxic effects in animals. A hydrogenated preparation of the three pure chemicals in ergotoxine, marketed under the trade name Hydergine, is now the most widely used agent for improving the mental functions of the elderly. Hydergine exerts a mild alerting action reminiscent of caffeine.

The twenty-fifth semisynthetic ergot Hofmann prepared by combining lysergic acid with different amines was lysergic acid diethylamide, abbreviated LSD-25. Sandoz pharmacologists, unimpressed with the compound's effects in animals, ceased development of this particular formulation. According to company policy, LSD-25 should therefore have been discarded and never synthe-

The Haight-Ashbury district of San Francisco in the 1960s was a gathering place for hippies and a focal point of drug-culture experimentation.

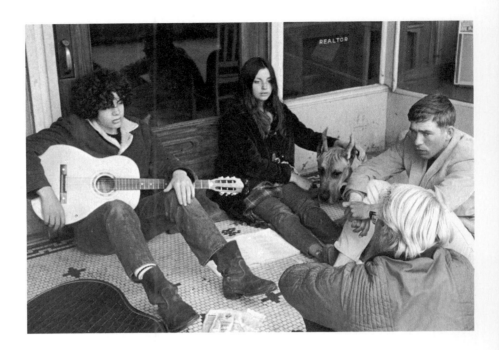

sized again. However, in 1943, acting under a "peculiar presentiment" that the compound possessed as yet undiscovered properties, Hofmann decided to synthesize it one more time.

This time, as he was completing the purification and crystallization of the LSD, Hofmann was overcome by some unusual sensations. The next day he wrote Arthur Stoll, who was his superior at Sandoz, a memorandum of the historic event: "Last Friday, April 16, 1943, I was forced to interrupt my work in the laboratory in the middle of the afternoon and proceed home, being affected by a remarkable restlessness combined with a slight dizziness. At home I lay down and sank into a not unpleasant intoxicated-like condition, characterized by an extremely stimulated imagination. In a dreamlike state with eyes closed I perceived an uninterrupted stream of fantastic pictures, extraordinary shapes with intense, kaleidoscopic play of colors. After some two hours this condition faded away."

Hofmann thought his mental aberrations were probably caused by the chemical he had just finished synthesizing. He tested this supposition on April 19 by ingesting 0.25 milligrams of LSD-25, an amount that for most drugs would be regarded as an extremely small dose. We know now that, considering its potency, this is a massive dose of LSD. Not surprisingly, Hofmann's reactions were pronounced.

Everything in my field of vision wavered and was distorted as if seen in a curved mirror. . . . Pieces of furniture assumed grotesque, threatening forms. . . . The lady next door, whom I scarcely recognized, . . . was no longer Mrs. R. but rather a malevolent, insidious witch with a colored mask. . . . Even worse than the demonic transformations of the outer world were the alterations that I perceived in myself, in my inner being. Every exertion of my will, every attempt to put an end to the disintegration of the outer world and the dissolution of my ego, seemed to be wasted effort. A demon had invaded me, had taken possession of my body, mind and soul. I jumped up and screamed, trying to free myself from him, but then sank down again and lay helpless on the sofa. . . . I was siezed by the dreadful fear of going insane. I was taken to another world, another place, another time. My body seemed to be without sensation, lifeless, strange. Was I dying? Was this the transition? At times I believed my self to be outside my body, and then perceived clearly, as an outside observer, the complete tragedy of my situation. . . . Would [my wife and three children] ever understand that I had not experimented thoughtlessly, irresponsibly, but rather with the utmost caution, and that such a result was in no way foreseeable?"

Hofmann recovered in about fourteen hours. His colleagues at Sandoz could hardly believe what had happened. A few of them ingested small doses of LSD and confirmed everything that Hofmann had described. The company tried to find therapeutic, commercial utility for LSD. They provided free samples and financial support to many investigators. For example, LSD was investigated as a possible adjunct to psychotherapy, to help "make conscious the unconscious." Though some psychiatrists involved in this venture reported success, others felt that the sensory distortions and psychotomimetic effects interfered with therapy. Other practitioners tried giving single large doses of LSD to alcoholics, in hopes that an overwhelming psychedelic experience might shock the patient into becoming sober. There were initial reports of success, but subsequent, more detailed studies showed that treatment without LSD but with the same psychological and emotional support that had accompanied the LSD treatment produced similar results. LSD was also administered to terminal cancer patients to help them tolerate the intense pain and accept their fate. Again, the first investigators were enthusiastic, but subsequent researchers found that the patients' experiences included as many "bad trips" as good ones.

With the enormous popularization of LSD by Timothy Leary and other advocates in the 1960s, tragically adverse reactions began to be documented. Many people killed themselves because of illusory thoughts and perceptions prompted by the drug. In a number of instances LSD psychoses precipitated long-term schizophrenic breaks in people who might have gone through life in reasonably good psychological health but for their drug experience. Psychologists examining chronic users of LSD detected apparently irreversible impairment in the thinking processes of a significant proportion of the test sample.

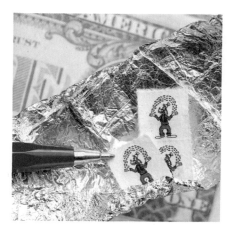

These LSD stamps contain doses of the homemade street drug.

Structures and uses of ergot drugs

Chemical structure   **Actions and uses**

Ergotamine

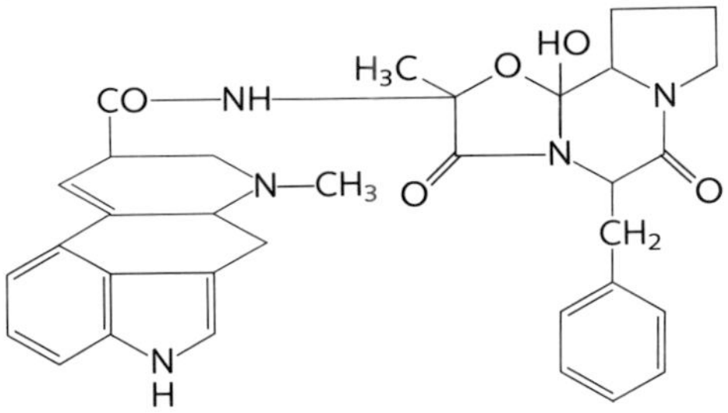

H₃C

CO—NH

N—CH₃

HO

N

N

O

CH₂

N
H

Vasoconstrictor
Uterine stimulant
In large doses, stimulates gastroin-
    testinal smooth muscle and con-
    stricts pupils
Blocks effects of norepinephrine

Ergocristine

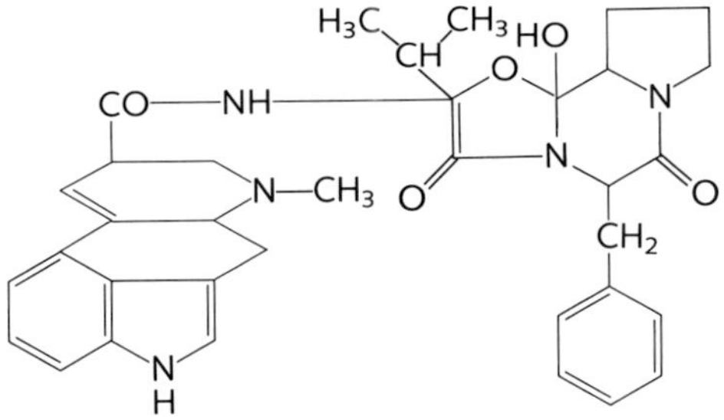

H₃C   CH₃ HO
CH

CO—NH

N—CH₃

N

N

O

CH₂

N
H

Vasoconstrictor
Uterine stimulant

Ergonovines

Ergonovine maleate

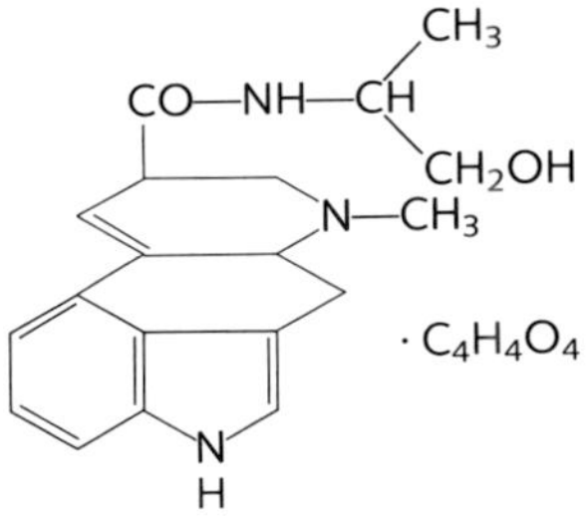

CH₃
CO—NH—CH
CH₂OH
N—CH₃

· C₄H₄O₄

N
H

Uterine stimulant
Reduces bleeding (contraction of
    uterus compresses bleeding ves-
    sels)

Chemical structure

Actions and uses

Methysergide maleate

C₂H₅

Blocks serotonin receptors
Prevents migraine

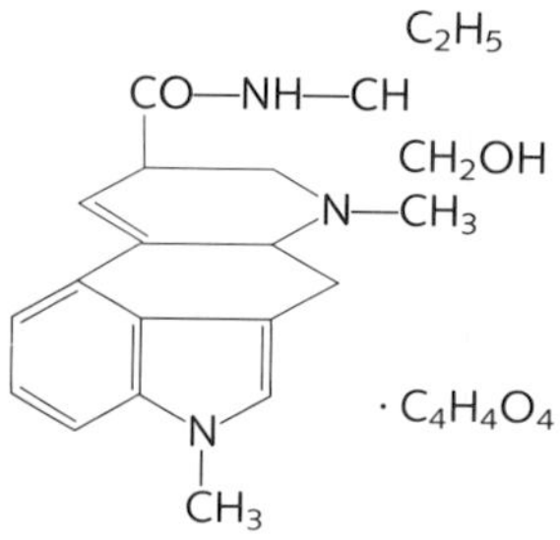

· C₄H₄O₄

Lysergic acid diethylamide (LSD)

Limited use in psychiatry

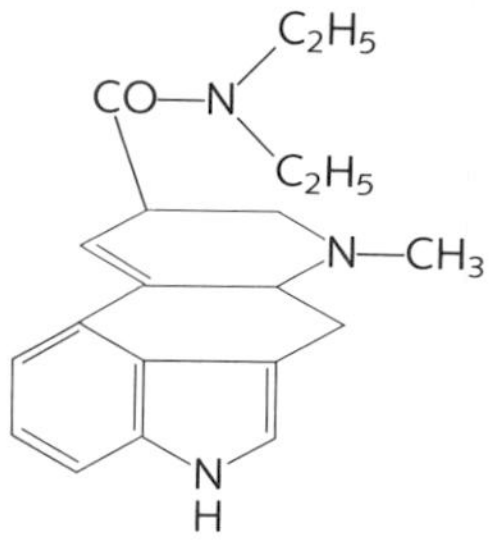

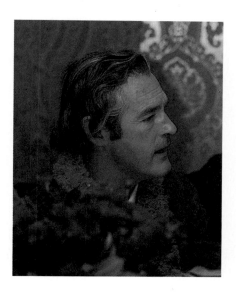

With so much adverse publicity, governments throughout Europe and North America imposed progressively harsh restrictions on the use of LSD, even for research purposes. Today, almost no LSD research is conducted in human subjects.

How Psychedelics Work

All the major psychedelic drugs bear a close chemical resemblance to the neurotransmitters serotonin, norepinephrine, and dopamine. Two of the four rings in LSD's chemical structure are identical to the ring system in serotonin, and the side chain attached to the ring structure of serotonin is identical to another

Timothy Leary (1920–   ), photographed in San Francisco around the time he was first popularizing LSD.

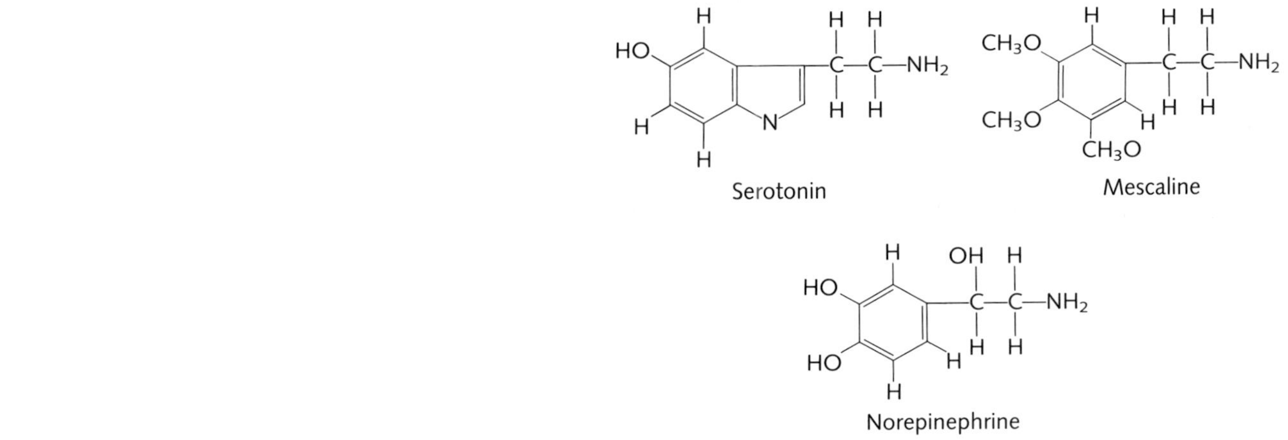

Serotonin Mescaline

Norepinephrine

part of the LSD molecule. The chemical structure of mescaline is closer to that of norepinephrine or dopamine, but careful examination also reveals some similarities to serotonin (see the chemical structures above), while psilocin and psilocybin and yet another psychedelic compound called dimethyltryptamine, or DMT, are such close chemical relatives of serotonin that it would seem only reasonable to assume their actions must have something to do with that neurotransmitter.

In spite of these impressive structural similarities, however, it has proved quite difficult to pinpoint exact mechanisms by which psychedelic drugs might affect norepinephrine, serotonin, and dopamine transmission. In 1953, not long after LSD was first described by Albert Hofmann, another drug scientist,

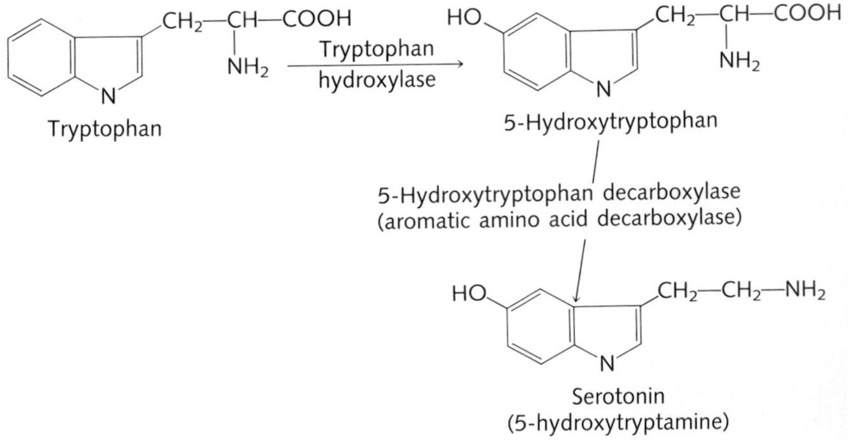

Tryptophan

Tryptophan hydroxylase

5-Hydroxytryptophan

5-Hydroxytryptophan decarboxylase (aromatic amino acid decarboxylase)

Serotonin (5-hydroxytryptamine)

In two enzyme-mediated operations, tryptophan is converted to serotonin.

the British pharmacologist John Gaddum, conducted experiments that suggested one hypothetical mechanism of action, but other researchers just as rapidly noted contradictions. Gaddum had been measuring the ability of serotonin to contract the uterus. It does this, in rather low concentrations, by acting at specific serotonin receptors, which is why some researchers feel that the body's natural serotonin takes part in the normal process of labor and delivery. Gaddum observed that low concentrations of LSD blocked the effects of serotonin upon the uterus, and on the assumption that serotonin receptors in the brain are similar to those in the uterus, he speculated that LSD exerts its psychedelic actions by blocking serotonin receptors in the brain. Subsequent investigators tested this hypothesis by examining a series of LSD derivatives—some of which block serotonin receptors and some of which do not—and comparing their psychedelic effects. 2-Bromo LSD, whose chemical structure differs only slightly from that of LSD, proved even more potent than LSD in blocking serotonin-induced contractions of the uterus but produced no psychedelic effects in humans, even in fairly high doses. This seemed to be rather strong evidence that Gaddum was wrong. Another apparent contradiction to Gaddum's theory was that mescaline, while an effective psychedelic drug, is not a serotonin antagonist.

In more recent years, researchers have examined the actions of psychedelic drugs directly in the brain, utilizing microelectrodes to record the firing rate of

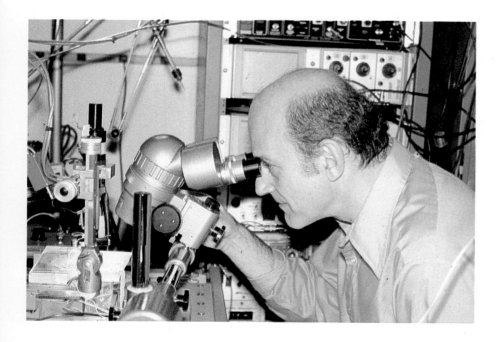

George Aghajanian (1932–   ) at the apparatus he uses to record the activity of single serotonin (and other) neurons in rat brain slices. The brain tissue is kept alive in a special chamber of the apparatus. A microelectrode can be guided into the dorsal raphe nucleus, where the serotonin neurons are located. The apparatus can then record the effects of any drugs and neurotransmitters that the experimenter introduces into the solution perfusing the tissue.

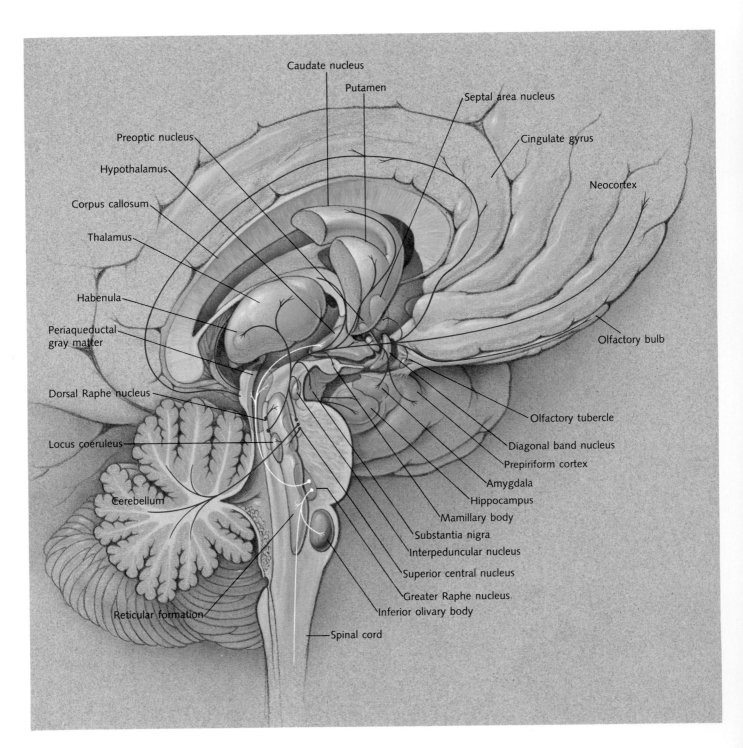

Caudate nucleus

Putamen

Septal area nucleus

Cingulate gyrus

Neocortex

Preoptic nucleus

Hypothalamus

Corpus callosum

Thalamus

Habenula

Periaqueductal gray matter

Olfactory bulb

Dorsal Raphe nucleus

Locus coeruleus

Cerebellum

Reticular formation

Spinal cord

Olfactory tubercle

Diagonal band nucleus

Prepiriform cortex

Amygdala

Hippocampus

Mamillary body

Substantia nigra

Interpeduncular nucleus

Superior central nucleus

Greater Raphe nucleus

Inferior olivary body

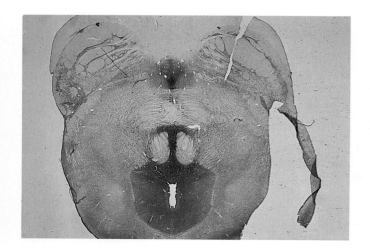 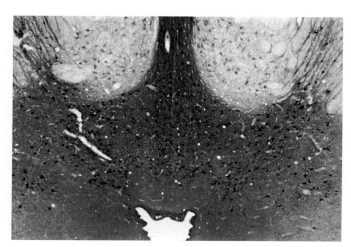

individual neurons. George Aghajanian, at Yale University, has been one of the pioneers in using this method to record the activities of serotonin-containing neurons. It is a technique well suited to the unique anatomical distribution of these neurons.

In the same classic studies of the mid-1960s in which Swedish investigators Kjell Fuxe and Annica Dahlström mapped norepinephrine and dopamine neurons in the brain (see Chapter 5), these two scientists also worked out the pathways for serotonin. They found that all the serotonin projections in the brain originate from a group of nuclei in the midline of the brainstem. These are called the raphe nuclei, from the Greek word describing a seamlike union of two halves, which is just what the raphe nuclei resemble. The serotonin cells in the raphe nuclei give rise to axons that ascend and ramify all over the brain, but with particularly dense projections in the limbic system. Because the cell bodies of all the serotonin neurons are so compactly clustered, microelectrodes inserted into neuronal cells in the raphe nucleus are certain to measure the activity of cells that contain serotonin, as opposed to any other type of neurotransmitter.

Aghajanian injected rats with small doses of LSD and then recorded the electrical activity of serotonin cells in the animals' raphe nuclei. His electrical tracings showed that LSD caused the serotonin neurons to abruptly stop firing (see the tracing on page 201). This effect was all the more impressive because only very low doses of LSD were required and no other neuronal cells in the vicinity of the raphe nuclei responded in the same way. Some of the other psychedelic drugs, including psilocybin, psilocin, and dimethyltryptamine, produced the same effect as LSD, but Aghajanian was disappointed to find that certain psychedelic compounds did not. Mescaline, for example did not consis-

Dorsal raphe nucleus in monkey brainstem, viewed at two magnifications. These cells are the main source of serotonin in the forebrain of the monkey and are very similar to human serotonin cells. *Left* A slice through the entire midbrain of a monkey. *Right* Higher magnification of the portion that contains serotonin cell bodies (the darkly stained spots are individual serotonin nerve cells). The two large, pale clusters are cells that control eye movements and do not contain serotonin.

Facing page Serotonin pathways in the brain.

Right Serotonin cells from a raphe nucleus in a rat's brainstem, labeled by a red fluorescent dye attached to a serotonin antibody. *Below* Serotonin nerve fibers in the cerebral cortex of a monkey, shown at two different magnifications. These photographs are from the part of the cortex necessary for the perception of touch. Serotonin nerve fibers arise primarily from cells in the raphe nuclei and spread extensively throughout the cerebral cortex. They are more abundant and more highly differentiated in primates (including humans and monkeys) than in lower species of animals.

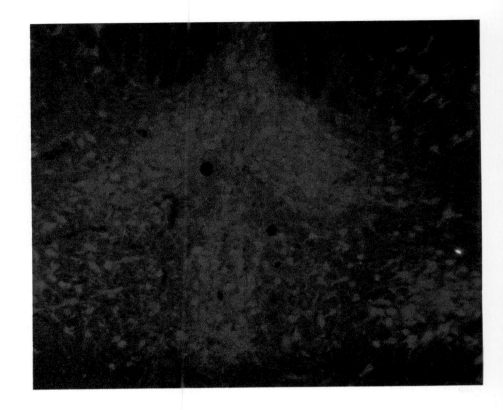

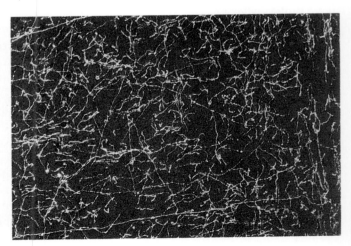

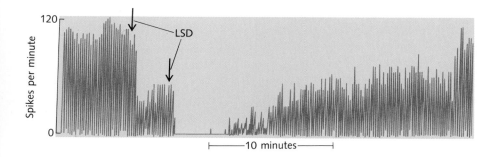

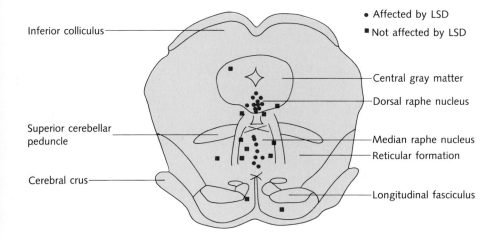

Inferior colliculus

Superior cerebellar
peduncle

Cerebral crus

● Affected by LSD
■ Not affected by LSD

Central gray matter

Dorsal raphe nucleus

Median raphe nucleus

Reticular formation

Longitudinal fasciculus

Top Effect of LSD on raphe neuron firing. The normal activity of dorsal raphe neurons, approximately 120 spikes per minute, is represented at the left of this recording (obtained using the apparatus illustrated on page 197). A first administration, of 10 micrograms per kilogram of LSD, causes the firing to slow, and a second administration, of 5 micrograms per kilogram, stops the raphe neurons from firing altogether. The neurons recover gradually, returning to normal activity over a period of about 20 minutes. *Bottom* Section through the midbrain of a rat showing sites affected by LSD and sites where either no effect is noted or where LSD causes firing to accelerate rather than to cease. The only neurons whose firing slows are the serotonin-containing neurons of the raphe nucleus.

tently slow the firing of raphe cells. Moreover, lisuride, an LSD derivative that has no psychedelic actions at fairly high doses in humans, was just as potent as LSD in stopping the raphe cells from firing.

In more recent studies, Aghajanian has focused not on the serotonin neurons of the raphe nuclei but on the norepinephrine neurons of the locus coeruleus. As we saw in Chapter 6, the locus coeruleus cell bodies give rise to axons that ramify all over the brain and provide the majority of the norepinephrine neuronal input in most brain regions. Amphetamine releases norepinephrine from these nerve terminals by displacing the norepinephrine from the neurotransmitter storage vesicles. Presumably, the overall influence of amphetamine on brain function is therefore somewhat different than what occurs when the locus coeruleus fires rapidly. The amphetamine-induced seepage of norepinephrine out of nerve terminals probably elicits a milder type of activa-

Electrical stimulation of locus coeruleus neurons causes repeated release of norepinephrine (N) and rapid firing of adjacent postsynaptic neurons. This effect is probably more intense than that of amphetamines (A), which act by displacing norepinephrine from its storage vesicles in the ends of locus coeruleus, among other, neurons.

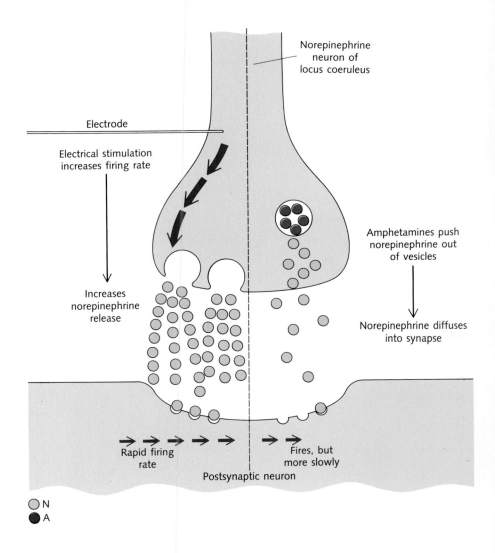

Norepinephrine neuron of locus coeruleus

Electrode

Electrical stimulation increases firing rate

Amphetamines push norepinephrine out of vesicles

Increases norepinephrine release

Norepinephrine diffuses into synapse

Rapid firing rate

Fires, but more slowly

Postsynaptic neuron

○ N
● A

tion than does the repetitive and presumably more robust ejection of norepinephrine that occurs with rapid firing of the locus coeruleus. Drug-induced changes in animal behavior support this conceptual model. Amphetamine elicits behavioral activation, represented by the rats or mice running about the cage. In contrast, electrical stimulation of the locus coeruleus produces a more dramatic startle response. It is difficult to observe a rat and make inferences about what the animal is feeling, but rats in whom the locus coeruleus has been stimulated seem to go into a state of panic. They stare about, hyper-responsive to all stimuli in the environment, whether visual, auditory, or tactile.

Rats show the same hyper-responsiveness to environmental stimuli—jumping abruptly at the sound of fingers snapping or in response to a puff of air in the face—when they have been treated with a psychedelic drug. And as you will recall, hyper-responsiveness to sensory stimuli of all modalities is just what one observes in humans under the influence of psychedelic drugs. Attracted by the similarity between the behavior of rats on LSD and their reaction to stimulation of the locus coeruleus, Aghajanian embarked in 1980 upon a series of studies to evaluate how psychedelic drugs affect the locus coeruleus. He showed that any kind of sensory stimulation—sight, sound, smell, taste, or tactile sensation—speeds up the firing of locus coeruleus neurons in rats, and that the accelerated firing is greatly enhanced by treating the animals with LSD or mescaline. In contrast, nonpsychedelic drugs, such as amphetamines and antidepressants, fail to exert this effect. Moreover, the LSD analogue methysergide, which has no psychedelic effects in humans, is correspondingly ineffective in enhancing the reactivity of locus coeruleus neurons to sensory stimulation.

Although psychedelic drugs increase the response of locus coeruleus cells to sensory stimulation, they do not cause the neurons to fire spontaneously in the absence of such stimulation. Moreover, directly applying LSD or mescaline to locus coeruleus neurons does not enhance the neurons' response to sensory stimulation. We must therefore conclude that the effect of psychedelic drugs on sensory stimulation is indirect—the drugs presumably interact with a different set of neurons that in turn make direct contact with the locus coeruleus.

What is particularly fascinating about Aghajanian's findings is how nicely they correspond to what we know about the effects of psychedelic drugs in humans, and how readily they explain the way psychedelic drugs accentuate all our sensory perceptions. The locus coeruleus is a funneling mechanism that integrates all sensory input. Viewed in this way, the observations of Aghajanian can explain synesthesia. If the locus coeruleus lumps all types of sensory messages—from sights, sounds, tactile pressures, smells, tastes—into a generalized excitation system within the brain, one can readily appreciate that stimulation of the locus coeruleus will cause the drug user to feel that sensations are crossing the boundaries between different modalities.

Aghajanian's research may also illuminate how LSD influences the user's sense of self. The greatly accelerated firing of the locus coeruleus presumably provokes a powerful, patterned release of norepinephrine from nerve terminals throughout the brain. As we discussed earlier, the consequent alerting action would be much more pronounced than what occurs with the far more gradual leaking out of norepinephrine produced when amphetamine displaces the transmitter from the storage vesicles. This extremely enhanced level of alertness might possibly account for the "transcendent" mental state produced by psychedelic drugs. In other words, in a state of such heightened awareness, the drug user may become conscious of an "inner self" to which he or she is normally oblivious.

The effect of psychedelic drugs on locus coeruleus neurons is probably indirect, mediated by another, as yet unidentified group of sensory neurons.

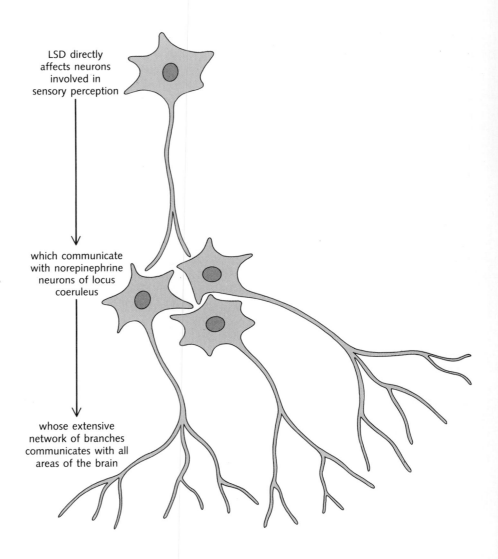

LSD directly affects neurons involved in sensory perception

which communicate with norepinephrine neurons of locus coeruleus

whose extensive network of branches communicates with all areas of the brain

As the investigation of psychedelic drug actions has taught us, sorting out the mechanism of action of drugs in the brain is not an altogether straightforward process. The pharmacologist may detect biochemical and electrophysiological effects of drugs, some of them rather potent. However, before concluding that a particular effect explains the clinical actions of the drug, the investigator must show that the most potent drugs in terms of clinical effect exhibit the same relative potency in terms of the observed biochemical or physiological effect. Drugs that fail to cause the physiological or biochemical action should also fail to produce the relevant clinical action.

Though the effects of psychedelic substances on the locus coeruleus are impressive, they may not fully explain the drugs' actions. Very recent research in numerous laboratories has revealed that psychedelic agents do exert potent effects on a serotonin receptor subtype, designated S_2. At S_2 receptors, psychedelic drugs mimic the effects of serotonin. The relative strengths with which psychedelic drugs influence S_2 receptors parallel the drugs' relative psychedelic potencies in humans. By influencing neurons with S_2 receptors, which have connections to the locus coeruleus, psychedelic drugs may indirectly change the firing of cells in the locus coeruleus.

Whether effects on the locus coeruleus and on serotonin S_2 receptors are closely linked in eliciting a psychedelic experience or whether one effect is more important than the other is as yet unclear, but whatever the answer may be, the research into the actions of psychedelic drugs has already enriched our understanding of how the brain regulates behavior. Apparently, norepinephrine neurons play an important role in regulating our general behavioral response to sensory stimulation. This response mechanism is quite different from other brain systems that are responsible for sensation per se. As explained in Chapter 6, the exclusively sensory systems of our brains, the systems responsible for vision, hearing, touch, and so on, are organized into precise point-to-point connections that enable us to scan the environment and assemble an almost photographic register of the scene in our brain. The pervasive ramifications of the locus coeruleus neuronal system, on the other hand, provide the emotional coloring, the feeling response, to sensory percepts. The research on psychedelic drugs also suggests that the amazing sense of oneness with the universe produced by psychedelic drugs might reflect an extreme activation of the locus coeruleus which causes a breakdown of the barriers between self and nonself. By influencing our level of awareness under normal circumstances, the locus coeruleus may play an important role in defining what psychologists call the ego, the awareness we each have of being a distinct person, separate from all others, confronting the universe on our own.

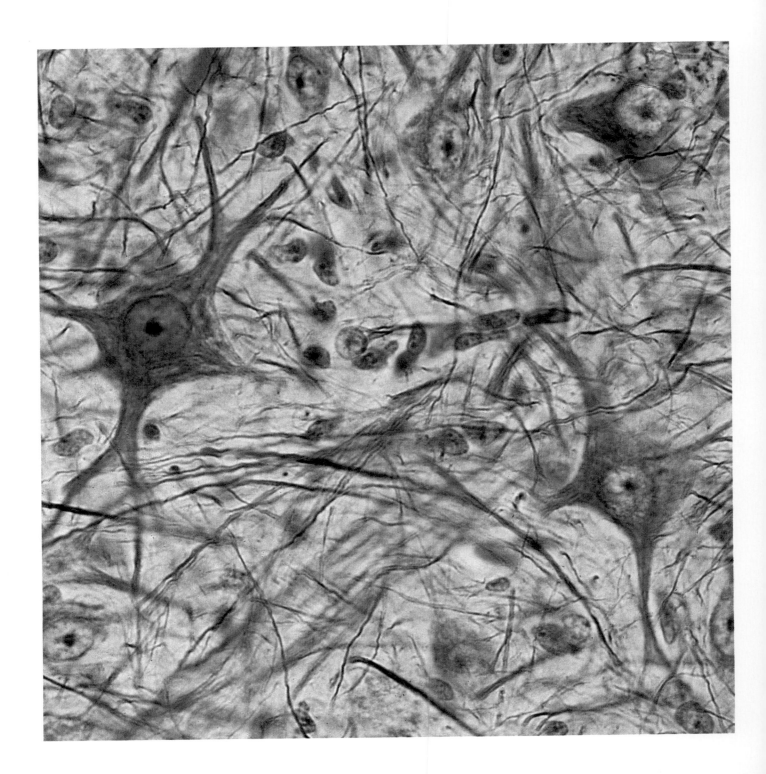

8 | Prospects

In this book I have tried to describe what modern neurotransmitter research is currently revealing about the actions of the principal drugs that influence the brain. I must emphasize, however, that, while the mechanisms described herein are either currently accepted theories or likely hypotheses, readers would be wrong to consider them ironclad certainties. In science, one never "proves" a theory. After initial experiments provide data suggesting a particular hypothesis, such as that antidepressants act by facilitating effects of norepinephrine and serotonin, further experiments are conducted to test the hypothesis. For instance, one might challenge the antidepressant hypothesis by destroying the norepinephrine and serotonin neurons in the brain and then administering antidepressants to see whether destruction of those neurons disrupts the drugs' ability to act. If such experiments seem to bear the hypothesis out, the results are said to "support" the hypothesis, not to prove that the hypothesis is a fact. These principles are universal in science, from the so-called hard sciences of physics and chemistry to the relatively less rigorous area of drug research.

Although we cannot describe drug actions in terms of incontrovertible fact, we can nevertheless state with some confidence that the vast amount of research done on psychoactive drugs has clarified a great deal about how they act and how the brain is organized. It is probably fair to add that the mechanisms for psychoactive drug actions are as well understood as the actions of almost any other class of drugs. Again, we do not know for *certain* exactly how the brain regulates specific behaviors, but we can formulate some educated guesses, and as long as they stand up to the trials we devise to test them, we can use these educated guesses as the bases for the next important advances in understanding.

Early on in this volume, we saw how the discovery of opiate receptors and the enkephalins revealed some aspects of the brain system that regulates pain perception and feeling states. Because emotions are very complicated mental

Facing page Central gray matter of the human spinal cord, magnified 160 times. Gold impregnation makes the neurons appear brown, while a toluidine counter-stain causes surrounding tissue to appear blue.

events, neurologists more or less expected to discover that other neurotransmitter systems are also involved in the modulation of feelings. They were therefore far from surprised when research with the antidepressants showed that norepinephrine and serotonin also influence mood. As yet, we can only guess at how the enkephalin and the amine neurotransmitter roles may differ. Perhaps the best evidence we have so far consists of the known effects of the drugs in humans. The euphoric state produced by opiates is a passive, dreamy affair. Individuals under the influence of opiate drugs seem immersed in a blissful reverie that is nevertheless readily distinguished from the somnolence produced by the same drugs. On the other hand, antidepressants imbue the recovering depressive with an exhuberant well-being that motivates the patient to resume normal life activities. Stimulants such as amphetamine and cocaine seem to exert an even more direct and invigorating influence on behavior.

Research psychiatrists attempting to dissect the actions of antidepressants have had a hard time distinguishing between actions mediated by norepinephrine and actions mediated by serotonin. Most antidepressants influence both neurotransmitters, but some of these drugs are more norepinephrine-specific and others have a greater effect on serotonin. For instance, chemists have synthesized drugs that inhibit serotonin but not norepinephrine uptake, and vice versa. Certain psychiatrists who have looked carefully at the clinical effects of the more selective antidepressants speculate that serotonin and norepinephrine are involved in different types of mood systems. These researchers suggest that facilitating norepinephrine transmission produces an energizing influence, spurring the user into action. This is also descriptive of the feelings brought on by cocaine and amphetamine, which act predominantly upon norepinephrine and have a lesser influence on serotonin. On the other hand, serotonin may be important in promoting a generalized sense of well-being. If these speculations are valid, it would seem most helpful to a depressed patient to enhance the activities of both neurotransmitters. Interestingly, of various antidepressants that have been employed, the most consistently effective are those that do act to a comparable extent upon both the norepinephrine and the serotonin systems.

Thus, while norepinephrine and serotonin both influence mood-regulating systems in the brain, each has a different role in influencing behavior. There are probably a number of other neurotransmitters besides those we have just mentioned—enkephalin, norepinephrine, and serotonin—participating in the regulation of mood. As we saw in Chapter 1, the number of known neurotransmitters exceeds fifty, and the total number in the brain is likely to be in excess of one hundred. Accordingly, the notion that many distinct mood molecules may be operating in our nervous system is not at all farfetched.

The antischizophrenic actions mediated by drugs that block dopamine receptors and the exacerbation of schizophrenic symptoms mediated by amphetamines, which release dopamine, all point to one transmitter. These facts enable us to make certain speculations about the normal role of dopamine in the brain. The major schizophrenic symptoms controlled by neuroleptic drugs are delusions (false ideas) and hallucinations (false sensory perceptions), so perhaps dopamine is one of the components of a neurological system designed to keep our thoughts and perceptions in accord with the reality of our environment. Perhaps without appropriate dopamine neuronal functioning we would be incapable of sorting through the jumble of thoughts and perceptions that assault us, unable to determine which of them are consonant with the real world and which are products of our own inner musings. The hypothesis that the dopamine system sorts the "wheat" from the "chaff" fits with what is known about the mental state of psychiatric patients undergoing an acute schizophrenic decompensation. At a certain critical stage in each schizophrenic episode, these patients are in contact with reality but feel overwhelmed by a barrage of terrifying thoughts. Psychosis supervenes when the patients resolve this muddle by adopting a new set of concepts—their delusions—and attending to their auditory hallucinations as if the voices were really there. Many research psychiatrists feel that neuroleptics relieve the pressure of the schizophrenic patients' frightening thoughts. In some cases, the drug seems to help patients recognize that their delusions are false. In other cases, patients may fail to achieve that insight, but under the influence of the drug they feel less compelled to heed the delusions or hallucinations. Thanks to the antischizophrenic drugs, patients are no longer obliged to work out a psychotic solution to protect themselves from total disintegration.

The actions of benzodiazepines imply that GABA is the neurotransmitter most closely linked to anxiety. Presumably, the benzodiazepine- and GABA-receptor machinery are part of a physiological system that, when disordered, gives rise to a fear response in the absence of a threat in the environment. (As we saw in Chapter 6, one clue to the meaning of anxiety may be the similarity between anxiety and fear.) Suppose there were a brain system that regulated our emotional status along a placidity-anxiety continuum. Extremes would be unhealthy. A person who was overly placid would have little motivation to do anything, while a person who was excessively anxious might be too paralyzed to act effectively. Perhaps the properly functioning GABA system prepares the organism to deal with perceived threats, a biologically important normal response whose derangement results in a debilitating excess of anxiety. We must remember, however, that GABA is the most abundant neurotransmitter in the brain, present in almost fifty times the number of neurons as contain norepinephrine, serotonin, or the enkephalins, and therefore it is probably involved in many brain functions besides the regulation of anxiety.

The last group of drugs we examined, the psychedelic drugs, produce a profoundly altered state of consciousness. Unlike the hallucinations of the schizophrenic, the "visions" brought on by psychedelic drugs consist primarily of a subjectively enhanced perception of the environment with some attendant distortions. Similarly, alterations in thought processes under the influence of psychedelic drugs do not involve grossly psychotic, aberrant ideas. Instead, the drug user feels that he or she is "more conscious." Many proselytizers for psychedelic drugs have argued that these agents produce a heightened level of awareness and reveal a world of the mind that is "more real" than what we normally experience. Of course, whether one considers psychedelic drugs to produce enhanced and "good" or distorted and "bad" awareness is a matter of value judgment as well as evaluation of scientific data. What is important is that research into the mechanism of these effects suggests that one small nucleus in the brain, the locus coeruleus, may be responsible for the intensity with which we color our thoughts and sensations. Since the locus coeruleus is such a discrete structure, it may be more amenable to research than many of the other, more diffuse brain systems influenced by drugs.

Through all we have discussed in this and other chapters, a theme recurs. Drugs produce remarkable influences upon the brain, some resulting in altered mental states that men and women may pursue for recreational purposes, others being of considerable importance in the treatment of emotional distress. Understanding how these drugs act at a molecular level has greatly enhanced pharmacologists' ability to develop new more potent, more selective, and safer drugs, on the one hand by giving drug developers more control over the specific action of a drug at receptor sites, and on the other hand by contributing to the ongoing discovery of neurotransmitters which can either be put to therapeutic use themselves or become new targets for drug therapy.

As we have seen in the preceding chapters, the stories of most of the major therapeutic drugs presently employed in psychiatry are largely tales of serendipity. Now that pharmacologists are learning how these agents act biochemically, however, they are developing techniques that will almost literally sculpt new drugs to fit their intended sites of action with far greater strength and selectivity than the parent drugs whose discoveries were accidental.

Conventional techniques for screening new drugs in the pharmaceutical industry have generally utilized intact animals. To seek out a new antiepileptic drug, for example, a researcher might pretreat a series of rats with various test chemicals, connect wires to the rats' skulls, and turn on an electric current to produce convulsions. If one of the chemicals appears to block the electrically induced convulsions, that substance becomes a candidate for further development; and if, after further testing, the drug is targeted for the marketplace, laboratory chemists will attempt to modify its chemical structure in order to improve its potency and selectivity.

When the only drug-screening procedures available are tests in intact animals, improving on the initial structure of a drug is quite a difficult proposition. To understand why, let us suppose that a chemist has synthesized a number of related chemicals, four of which demonstrate high pharmacological potency. One of those four chemicals may be more potent simply because it is not so rapidly metabolized in the liver. Another may be more potent because it is more easily absorbed from the stomach and intestine into the bloodstream. A third may penetrate more readily from the blood into the brain. Finally, the fourth may be more potent because of its actions at the receptor site. These differences in drug activity are very difficult to identify by observing changes in intact animals. In contrast, when the techniques invented by neuroscientists to discover neurotransmitter receptors are adapted for use in psychoactive drug development—techniques that can measure receptor-binding in a test tube— then the drug-screening process becomes much more informative.

The new drug-screening techniques are also more efficient. An adequate screening in intact animals may require 25,000 milligrams of the chemical under study. The task of synthesizing this amount of drug could occupy the chemist for a month. Test-tube analysis of the same chemical's behavior at receptors can be accomplished with a tenth of a milligram, an amount that can be prepared in a couple of days.

Once the pharmacologist has determined the relative potencies of several chemical agents at a receptor site, it is easy to draw inferences concerning which variations in molecular structure enhance the ability of the drug to interact with the receptor site. Thus, the subsequent generation of test drugs can be designed to interact with receptors more efficiently and are therefore likely to exhibit a much higher absolute potency. Repetition of this strategy— by analyzing and imitating the chemical structures of the most potent second-generation drugs—can eventually result in an enhancement of drug potency by several thousandfold.

A more potent drug is by definition more selective. That is, it binds so specifically and preferentially at its target receptor that it produces its thera- peutic effects even when administered in extremely low doses. Because most side effects are produced when a drug binds to sites other than the specific receptor or enzyme where it exerts its therapeutic actions, a drug potent enough to be administered in very low doses is less likely to elicit any but the one desired pharmaceutical action. When doses of a potent drug are just high enough to influence the site of therapeutic action, the drug concentrations will be much too low to affect sites responsible for side effects.

In the very first chapter, when we discussed the role of acetylcholine in Alzheimer's disease, we saw how neurotransmitter studies influence more than just the screening of new drugs. The continuing advances in our understanding of neurotransmitter systems can be expected to reveal many new neurotrans- mitters that may in turn suggest strategies for the *development* of novel drugs. As we saw in Chapter 2, research on the enkephalins and related peptides sparked a great interest in the search for and analysis of peptide neurotransmit- ters. Of the large number of newly discovered peptide neurotransmitters char- acterized since 1975, almost all are confined to neuronal pathways of the brain in as discrete and interesting a fashion as the enkephalins. Some are highly concentrated in areas involved in emotional regulation. Others are located in brain nuclei that have been implicated in particular types of perception or cognition. Most of these transmitters have been discovered so recently that no new drugs have yet been developed to influence them selectively, but continued research is likely to result in drugs whose actions are just as remarkable as the antischizophrenic, antidepressant, and antianxiety drugs already employed in clinical practice. Particularly tantalizing is the possibility that drugs acting discretely upon some of the newly discovered transmitters will exert effects unlike any produced by the drugs we know today, modulating mental function in a far more subtle and precise manner than is now conceivable and thus altering individual psychological symptoms in a highly selective fashion. At the very least, we can expect future drugs to be free of the side effects that hamper the use of drugs currently available to psychiatry.

As new drug agents are developed, they too, like the opiates, neuroleptics, and other psychoactive drugs before them, will be used as probes to clarify brain function in health and disease. Brain research of the past decade, especially the study of neurotransmitters, has proceeded at a furious pace, achieving progress equal in scope to all the accomplishments of the preceding fifty years—and the pace of discovery continues to accelerate. The final years of the twentieth century may witness unparalleled advances in our understanding of the brain and, even more exciting, in our ability to put this understanding to therapeutic use.

Recommended Readings

Akil, H., Watson, S. J., Young, E., Lewis, M. E., Khachaturian, H., Walker, J. M., Endogenous opioids: Biology and function, *Annual Review of Neuroscience,* 7:223–255, 1984. A thorough review.

Bleuler, E., *Dementia Praecox or the Group of Schizophrenias,* International Universities Press, New York, 1950. The classic definition of schizophrenia.

Bloom, F. E., The endorphins: A growing family of pharmacologically pertinent peptides, *Annual Review of Pharmacology and Toxicology,* 23:151–170, 1983. An integration of research about opiate-like peptides.

Cooper, J. R., Bloom, F. E., Roth, R. H., *The Biochemical Basis of Neuropharmacology,* 4th ed., Oxford University Press, New York, 1982. The best basic explanation of the chemical systems upon which drugs exert their effects.

Davis, J. M., Maas, J. W., (eds.), *The Affective Disorders,* American Psychiatric Press, Washington, D.C., 1983. A useful overview.

Greenblatt, D. J., Shader, R. I., Abernethy, D. R., Current status of benzodiazepines, *New England Journal of Medicine,* 308:354–358, 410–416, 1983. Covers all the clinical uses of benzodiazepines.

Grinspoon, L., Bakalar, J. B., *Cocaine,* Basic Books, New York, 1976. The best reference on the subject of cocaine.

Grinspoon, L., Bakalar, J., *Psychedelic Drugs Reconsidered,* Basic Books, New York, 1979. Puts these drugs in societal perspective.

Hofmann, A., *LSD: My Problem Child,* McGraw-Hill Book Company, New York, 1980. A personal account by the man who discovered LSD.

Kandel, E. R., Schwartz, J. H., *Principles of Neural Sciences,* 2d ed., Elsevier Publishing Company, New York, 1985. The best basic textbook on the brain.

Ray, O., *Drugs, Society and Human Behavior,* 3d ed., C. V. Mosby, St. Louis, 1983. An undergraduate text presenting psychoactive drugs in their historical and social contexts.

Snyder, S. H., *Madness and the Brain,* McGraw-Hill Book Company, New York, 1974. Deals with biological aspects of schizophrenia.

Snyder, S. H., *Biological Aspects of Mental Disorder,* Oxford University Press, New York, 1980. Reviews all the major psychiatric disorders.

Usdin, E., Skolnick, P., Tallman, J. F., Jr., Greenblatt, D., Paul, S. M., (eds.), *Pharmacology of Benzodiazepines,* MacMillan & Co., London, 1982. A collection of research articles on how benzodiazepines act.

Van Praag, H. M., Neurotransmitters and CNS disease: Depression, *Lancet,* 2:1259–1264, 1982. A concise review of biological features of depression.

Notes

pages 18–19
Table adapted from S. H. Snyder, *Biological Aspects of Mental Disorder*, Oxford University Press, New York, 1980, pp. 72–73.

page 29
Sydenham quote from O. S. Ray, *Drugs, Society and Human Behavior*, C. V. Mosby, St. Louis, 1972, p. 180.

page 30
T. De Quincey, *Confessions of an English Opium Eater*, E. P. Dutton, New York, 1907, p. 179.

page 31
Excerpted from D. I. Macht, The history of opium and some of its preparations and alkaloids, *Journal of the American Medical Association*, 64(6):477–481, February 1915.

pages 31–32
J. Jones, *The Mysteries of Opium Revealed*, Richard Smith, London, 1700, p. 32.

pages 33–34
M. A. Menges, A second report on the therapeutics of heroin, *New York Medical Journal*, 71(51):82–83, 1900.

page 45
Table adapted from S. H. Snyder, The opiate receptor, *American Journal of Psychiatry*, 135(6), June 1978.

page 63
Excerpted from E. Bleuler, *Dementia Praecox or the Group of Schizophrenias*, International University Press, New York, 1950, pp. 17, 34, 54.

page 64
Excerpted from J. D. Benjamin, A method for distinguishing and evaluating formal thinking disorders in schizophrenia, in J. S. Kasanin (ed.), *Language and Thought in Schizophrenia*, University of California Press, Berkeley, 1944, pp. 65–90.

page 65
Table adapted from S. H. Snyder, *Madness and the Brain*, McGraw-Hill, New York, 1974, p. 28.

pages 66–67
Excerpt from the American Psychiatric Association's *Diagnostic and Statistical Manual—III*, 3d ed., 1980, pp. 188–190.

page 83
Table adapted from I. Creese, M. W. Hamblin, S. E. Leff, D. R. Sibley, CNS dopamine receptors, in L. L. Iversen, S. D. Iversen, S. H. Snyder (eds.), *Handbook of Psychopharmacology*, Vol. 17, Plenum, New York, 1983, p. 88.

page 91
Plutarch quote from G. Zilboorg, *A History of Medical Psychology*, Norton, New York, 1941, p. 57.

page 92
Logan quote from R. R. Fieve, *Moodswing*, Bantam (in association with William Morrow), New York, 1975, pp. 29–30.

Tolstoy and Alvarez quotes from A. Alvarez, *The Savage God*, Random House, New York, 1972, pp. 222 and 267–268, 270.

V. Woolf, *A Writer's Diary*, L. Woolf (ed.), Harcourt Brace Jovanovich, New York, 1953, pp. 202–203.

page 93
S. Plath, *The Bell Jar*, Bantam (in association with Harper & Row), New York, 1971, p. 2.

J. Custance, *Wisdom, Madness and Folly*, Farrar, Straus, and Cudahy, New York, 1952.

pages 102–103
R. Kuhn, F. J. Ayd, Jr., B. Blackwell (eds.), in *Discoveries in Biological Psychiatry*, Lippincott, Philadelphia, 1970, p. 205.

page 123
S. H. Snyder, *Madness and the Brain*, McGraw-Hill, 1974, p. 172.

page 126
S. Freud, On the general effects of cocaine, *Medicinisch-chirurgisches Centralblatt*, 20:373–375, 1885.

page 127
Excerpted from S. Freud, Übër coca, *Centralblatt für dieges. Therapie*, 2:289–314, 1884, translated by S. A. Edminster; additions to translation by F. C. Redlich.

page 128
S. Freud, On the general effects of cocaine, *Medicinisch-chirurgisches Centralblatt*, 20:373–375, 1885.

page 131
R. R. Munroe, H. J. Drell, Use of stimulants obtained from inhalers, *Journal of the American Medical Association*, 135:909–910, 1937.

page 132
M. F. Lesses, A. Myerson, Correspondence, Benzedrine sulfate, *Journal of the American Medical Association*, 110:1507–1508, 1938.

T. Hemmi, How we handled the problem of drug abuse in Japan, in F. Sjoqvist, M. Tottie (eds.), *Abuse of Central Stimulants*, Raven Press, New York, 1969, p. 148.

pages 153–154
J. M. Da Costa, On irritable heart. A clinical study of a form of functional cardiac disorder and its consequences, *American Journal of Medical Science*, 61:17, 1871.

page 161
F. M. Berger, The use of antianxiety drugs, *Clinical Pharmacology and Therapeutics*, 29:291, 1981.

page 180
A. Huxley, *The Doors of Perception*, Harper & Row, New York, 1970, p. 16.

page 181
Ibid., pp. 22, 26, 55.

page 183
H. Osmond, A review of the clinical effects of psychotomimetic agents, *Annals of the New York Academy of Science*, March 14, 1957.

page 184
Hernández quote from O. S. Ray, *Drugs, Society and Human Behavior*, C. V. Mosby, St. Louis, 1972, p. 215.

page 188
A. Hofmann, *LSD: My Problem Child*, McGraw-Hill, New York, 1980, p. 103.

page 192
Ibid., p. 15.

page 193
Ibid., p. 17.

Sources of Illustrations

Paintings by Bill Andrews

facing page 1
© Biophoto Associates/Photo Researchers, Inc.

page 2
© A. Glauberman/Photo Researchers, Inc.

page 3
New York Academy of Medicine

page 4 (left and right)
© Arnold Kage/Peter Manfred, Inc.

page 6
After T. N. Jenkins, *Functional Mammalian Neuroanatomy,* 2d ed., Lea & Febiger, Philadelphia, 1978

page 9 (left)
Sanford L. Palay

page 9 (right)
© 1986 by SIU/Peter Arnold, Inc.

page 13
Adapted from M. J. Berridge, The molecular basis of communication within the cell, *Scientific American,* 253(4):144, October 1985

page 20
After W. A. Bain, Method of demonstrating humor transmission of effects of cardiac vagus stimulation in frogs, *Quarterly Journal of Experimental Physiology and*

Cognate Medical Sciences, 22:269–274, 1932, copyright with Sir Edward Sharpey Shafer's trustees.

page 24
Pamela Harper

page 25
Art Resource

page 26
Lynn Johnson/Black Star

page 28
Courtesy of Dr. Michael J. Kuhar and Dr. Errol B. Desouza

page 30
© A. B. Joyce/Photo Researchers, Inc.

page 30 (bottom)
The Granger Collection

page 32
© Mary Evans Picture Library/Photo Researchers, Inc.

page 33
Peter Arnold, Inc.

page 34 (top)
The Granger Collection

page 34 (bottom)
The Bettmann Archive

page 37
Adapted from S. H. Snyder, Opiate

receptors and internal opiates, *Scientific American,* 236(3):46, March 1977

page 40
Adapted from S. H. Snyder, Opiate receptors and internal opiates, *Scientific American,* 236(3):48, March 1977

page 41
Adapted from S. H. Snyder, Opiate receptors and internal opiates, *Scientific American,* 236(3):49, March 1977

page 42
Adapted from S. H. Snyder, Opiate receptors and internal opiates, *Scientific American,* 236(3):49, March 1977

page 44 (left)
Courtesy of Dr. Michael J. Kuhar and Dr. Errol B. Desouza

page 44 (right)
Courtesy of Dr. Michael J. Kuhar

page 50
After W. R. Martin, H. F. Fraser, A comparative study of physiological and subjective effects of heroin and morphine administered intravenously in post addicts, *Journal of Pharmacology and Experimental Therapeutics,* 133:388, 1961

page 52
After A. H. Beckett, Stereochemical factors in biological activities, *Fortschr. Arzneimittelforsch.,* 1:455, 1959

page 53
Adapted from S. H. Snyder, Opiate receptors and internal opiates, *Scientific American,* 236(3):53, March 1977

page 54
After J. Hughes, T. Smith, H. W. Kosterlitz, L. A. Fothergill, B. A. Morgan, H. R. Morris, Identification of two related pentapeptides from the brain with potent opiate agonist activity, *Nature,* 258:577–579, 1975

page 56
Adapted from S. H. Snyder, Opiate receptors and internal opiates, *Scientific American,* 236(3):52, March 1977

page 60
Derek Beyes/Life Picture Service

page 67
National Institutes of Health

page 68
Adapted from S. H. Snyder, Mending shattered minds, *Science Year* (World Book Encyclopedia), 1981, p. 135

page 69 (top)
Zalersky/Klemmer/Black Star

page 69 (bottom)
Jack Spratt/Black Star

page 71 (top)
Paris Medical, 134:453, Jul.–Dec. 1947

Page 71 (bottom)
New York Academy of Medicine

page 73
New York Botanical Garden

page 80
Adapted from S. H. Snyder, S. J. Peroutka, Relationship of neuroleptic drug effects at brain dopamine, serotonin, α-adrenergic and histamine receptors to clinical potency, *American Journal of Psychiatry,* 137(12):1520, December 1980

page 90
The Granger Collection

page 97
Courtesy of Dr. E. A. Zeller; from G. M. Everett, R. G. Wiegand, F. U. Rinaldi, Pharmacologic studies of some nonhydrazine MAO inhibitors, *Annals of the New York Academy of Science,* 107:1068, 1963

page 98 (bottom)
National Library of Medicine

Page 103 (bottom)
National Library of Medicine

page 107
© Dr. J. F. McGinty/Peter Arnold, Inc.

page 110
Adapted from L. Träskman, M. Åsberg, L. Bertilsson, L. Sjöstrand, Monoamine metabolites in CSF and suicidal behavior, *Archives of General Psychiatry,* 38:631–636, June 1981

page 114 (left)
UPI/Bettmann Newsphotos

page 114 (middle)
The Bettmann Archive, Inc.

page 114 (right)
UPI/Bettmann Newsphotos

page 115
Neuropsychobiology, 10:8, 1983

page 120
© Ellan Young/C. J. Collins/Photo Researchers, Inc.

page 122 (top)
© Allen Rokach/New York Botanical Garden

page 122 (bottom)
W. H. Hodge/© Peter Arnold, Inc.

page 123
The Bettmann Archive

page 124
Culver Pictures

page 125 (top)
W. H. Hodge/© Peter Arnold, Inc.

page 125 (bottom)
The Granger Collection

page 126
The Granger Collection

page 128
Arthur Tress/Photo Researchers, Inc.

page 129
Courtesy of the Alan Mason Chesnoy Medical Archives of Johns Hopkins Medical Institutions

page 131
Bruce Coleman, Inc.

page 132
© Bob Combs/Photo Researchers, Inc.

page 137
© Erika Stone

page 144 (top left and right; bottom)
Courtesy of Mark E. Molliver, M.D.

page 146
Courtesy of Mark E. Molliver, M.D.

page 150
The Granger Collection

page 160
Adapted from K. Rickels, R. W. Downing,
A. Winokur, Antianxiety drugs: Clinical
use in psychiatry, in L. L. Iversen, S. D.
Iversen, S. H. Snyder (eds.), *Handbook
of Psychopharmacology,* Vol. 13,
Plenum, New York, 1978, pp. 395–
430

page 164
Adapted from A. Goldstein, L. Aronow,
S. M. Kalman, *Principles of Drug Action,*
Harper & Row, New York, 1968,
p. 588

page 167
From R. E. Study, J. L. Barker, Cellular
mechanisms of benzodiazepine action,
*Journal of the American Medical
Association,* 247(15):2147–2151

page 168
Courtesy of Dr. Michael J. Kuhar

page 169
Adapted from C. Braestrup, R. F. Squires,
Pharmacological characterization of
benzodiazepine receptors in the brain,
European Journal of Pharmacology,
48:263–270, 1978

page 170 (left)
Adapted from J. F. Tallman, J. W. Thomas,
D. W. Gallager, GABAergic modulation
of benzodiazepine binding site sensitivity,
Nature, 274:383–385, 1978

page 170 (right)
Adapted from J. H. Skerritt, M. Willow,
G. A. R. Johnston, Diazepam
enhancement of low affinity GABA
binding to rat brain membranes,
Neuroscience Letters, 29:63–67, 1982

page 171 (left and right)
Courtesy of Dr. Michael J. Kuhar

page 178
Stephen Jennings

page 180
The Granger Collection

page 182
Gene Anthony/Black Star

page 184
© Paolo Koch/Photo Researchers, Inc.

page 185
© Michael Viard/Peter Arnold, Inc.

page 186 (left and right)
© Kal Muller 1977

page 189
The Botanical Museum, Harvard University

page 190
UPI/Bettmann Newsphotos

page 191
Leonard Lee Rue III

page 192
UPI/Bettmann Newsphotos

page 193
C. Fitch/Alpha

page 195
Gene Anthony/Black Star

page 197
Courtesy of G. K. Aghajanian, M.D.

page 199 (left and right)
Courtesy of Mark E. Molliver, M.D.

page 200 (top; bottom left and right)
Courtesy of Mark E. Molliver, M.D.

page 201 (top)
Adapted from G. K. Aghajanian, W. E. Foote,
M. H. Sheard, Action of psychotogenic
drugs on single midbrain raphe neurons,
*Journal of Pharmacology and
Experimental Therapeutics,* 171(2):181,
1970

page 201 (bottom)
Adapted from G. K. Aghajanian, W. E. Foote,
M. H. Sheard, Lysergic acid
diethylamide: Sensitive neuronal units in
the midbrain raphe, *Science,* 161:706–
708, 1968

page 206
Photo Researchers, Inc.

Index

Abstinence, 50, 51
Acetic acid, 19, 20
Acetyl coenzyme A, 19
Acetylcholine, 36, 103; and Alzheimer's disease, 24–27, 211; as model for neurotransmitters, 16–24
Acetylcholine pathways, 23
Acetylcholine receptors, 103
Acetylcholinesterase, 20, 21, 22, 26, 103
Adenylate cyclase, 12–13
Addiction, 2, 29, 41, 47–48, 95; to barbiturates, 156, 165; components of, 48–50; to morphine, 33, 128–129; to opiates, 33–34, 48–51; to opium, 30–32
Addictive potential: of barbiturates, 156; of benzodiazepines, 160, 161; of cocaine, 125, 126; of enkephalin derivatives, 59; of meprobamate, 158, 159; of opiates, 29
Adrenal gland, 87
Adrenaline, 130
Adverse drug reactions, 193–195
Affect (feeling state), 93, 118
Affective disorders, 93, 94, 113; amine hypothesis of, 111; environment in, 95
Affective system: effect of lithium on, 118–119
Aghajanian, George, 197, 198–201, 203
Agonists, 35–36, 39
Alcohol, 95, 129, 149, 156, 165, 166; action of, 173–174; depressive effects of, potentiated by benzodiazepines, 161, 177; inhibitory effects of GABA potentiated by, 166, 174
Alcoholics Anonymous, 51
Alcoholism, 51, 70, 95, 138; treatment of, 165, 193
Alertness: drug-induced, 203; from stimulants, 122, 126, 130, 131, 133, 135, 138, 148
Alles, Gordon, 131
Alvarez, A., 92
Alzheimer's disease, 24–27, 211
American Indians, 73, 185
"Amine hypothesis" (depression), 100, 103, 106–111
Amine neurotransmitters, 97, 100, 103, 107; and affective state, 118; in antidepressants, 111; deficiency of, in depression, 109; inactivation of, 103–106; and lag-time enigma, 111–112
Amine reuptake: inhibition of, 113F
Amine structures, 74
Amines, 208
Amino acid neurotransmitters, 106
Amino acids, 8–9, 52, 53, 176
Amphetamine abuse, 130–133, 135–136
Amphetamine psychosis, 138–140, 182
Amphetamines, 14, 30, 101, 119, 121–122, 203; action of, 149–149; chemical structure of, 136; effects of, 133–138, 201–202, 203, 208
Amygdala, 48, 84, 171
Analgesia, 2, 33, 41; search for non-addicting, 56–59

Anesthesia, 71; general, 129, 130; local, 7, 122, 127, 129–130

Angina, 36, 153

Anhalonium lewinii, 184

Animal models, 48, 50, 97; depression, 109, 111, 112

Animal studies, 3, 34, 41, 210–211; appetite suppressants, 135; benzodiazepines, 160–161, 166; drug-induced behavioral activation, 202–203; effect of chlorpromazine on brain dopamine, 77; iproniazid, 96–97; muscle relaxants, 158; pain perception, 44; psychedelic drugs, 190

Antagonists, 34–36, 39, 78

Antianxiety agents, 2, 159–177, 212

Antibody techniques, 55

Anticonvulsants, 174

Antidepressant drugs, 1–2, 14, 27, 98–100, 109, 203, 208, 212; action of, 117, 207; chemical structure of, 102; development of, 116; discovery of, 95–98; lag-time enigma, 111–112; second-generation, 111, 117; in treatment of anxiety, 152; *see also* Tricyclic antidepressants

Antihistamines, 71, 82

Antihypertensive drugs, 109

Antischizophrenic drugs, 1, 27, 59, 61–89, 96–97, 98, 101, 102, 109, 158, 208–209, 212; action of, 142, 148; development of, 116; in stimulant psychosis, 139, 140; *see also* Neuroleptic drugs

Anxiety, 62, 151–177; clinical picture of, 152–155; drugs in treatment of, 1, 2, 61, 128, 152; GABA and, 209; physical complaints in, 153–154; treatments for, 155–159

Anxiety neurosis, 153–154

Appetite suppression, 133, 135–136

Åsberg, Marie, 109–111

Asthma, 29, 130–131

Astrocytes, 4

ATP (*adenosine triphosphate*), 12

Atropa belladonna, 23, 24

Atropine, 24, 25, 36, 182

Attention deficit disorder, 137–138

Auditory hallucinations, 62, 138

Autism, 62–63

Awareness: psychedelics and, 203, 210

Axelrod, Julius, 104–106

Axonal conduction, 7

Axons, 4, 6, 8, 11, 142

Aztecs, 184

Bacteria: gram-negative, 157

Barbiturates, 1, 72, 73, 139, 149, 158–159, 160; actions and uses of, 156–157, 173–174; addiction to, 156, 165; binding sites, 175; chemical structure of, 162; depressive effects of, potentiated by benzodiazepines, 161, 177; effect on synaptic transmission, 164, 165, 166; inhibitory effects of GABA potentiated by, 166, 174; in treatment of anxiety, 156; in treatment of mania, 115

Barnard, Eric, 175

Basal nucleus, 22, 24–25

Bayer (drug co.), 33

Becquerel, Henri, 43

Behavior, human, 22, 204; neurotransmitter effects on, 208; peptide transmitters and, 56

Behavioral therapy, 155–156

Belladonna, 24

Benzedrine, 131, 132

Benzodiazepine receptors, 167–173, 174, 175

Benzodiazepines, 1, 149, 159–164; action of, 164–177, 209; binding sites, 175; inhibitory effect of GABA potentiated by, 166, 170, 174

Benzphetamine (Didrex), 134

Berger, Frank, 157–158, 161

Bernays, Martha, 126

Biochemical abnormalities (mental illness), 72, 151

Biochemical effect of drugs: antischizophrenic actions of iproniazid, 97–98 neuroleptics, 73, 74, 77, 83, 84; and therapeutic potential, 34–38, 42;

Biogenic amines, 74, 75, 76, 103; deficiency of, in depression, 109

Biologically determined illness, 65–68, 94–95; *see also* Genetic component

Bipolar affective disorder, 93, 94–95, 114, 117, 118

Bleuler, Eugen, 63–64

Blood-brain barrier, 26, 27, 59

Blood pressure, 14, 36, 73, 100–101, 109

Braestrup, Claus, 167–168

Brain, 1–27; anatomical divisions of, 17; concepts of, 7–8; effect of drugs on, 207–212; effect of stimulants on, 121–122, 140–149; locating opiate receptors in, 42–48; location of drug action in, 15–16; mechanism of drug action on, 204–205; natural "morphine" of, 51–59; organization and function of, 1, 3, 22, 27, 59, 88–89, 145, 177, 207–208; regulation of behavior, 205; regulation of emotions, 207–210, 211; selective action of drugs on, 157, 158–159

Brain cells, 3–7

Brain chemistry, 72, 74–75, 97, 100

Brain hemorrhage, 101

Brain membranes, 36, 38–39, 40, 82

Brain research, 1, 3, 35–36, 59, 84, 212

Brain strokes, 157

Brain structure: in pain perception, 43–48

Brain systems: for regulation of anxiety, 171–173

Brainstem, 47, 48, 84, 107, 199

Bretylium, 14

Brodie, Bernard, 74

Browning, Elizabeth Barrett, 31

Bupropion, 117

Burt, David, 82

Cade, John, 115–116

Caffeine, 121, 124, 125, 191

Cajal, Santiago Ramón y, 8

Cancer, 193

Candler, Asa, 125

Carbolines, 171–173

Carlsson, Arvid, 76–77, 78, 79, 83

Cell metabolism, 77

Cellular tolerance, 50

Cerebellum, 15–16, 142

Cerebral cortex, 4, 15, 36, 86, 142, 145, 146, 171; acetylcholine in, 22; and limbic system, 48

Chemical neurotransmission, 7; *see also* Neurotransmission

Chemical oscillator system (hypothesis), 118

Chemical probes, 1; amphetamines as, 122

Chemical substances: isolation of, from plant extracts, 126

Chemistry: of thinking and feeling, 3; *see also* Brain chemistry

Chen, K. K., 131

Childbirth, 190, 197
Chloride channels, 9–10
Chloride-ion channels, 174–176
Chlorpromazine, 70, 71–73, 158; clinical
    effects of, 74, 76, 78, 81, 82, 84;
    three-ring structure of, 101–102; in
    treatment of mania, 115; in treatment
    of schizophrenia, 96–97, 107–109
Choline, 19, 20–21, 25
Choline acetyltransferase, 19, 25
Christianity, 184–185
Churchill, Winston, 114
Ciba Drug Company, 73
Cingulate cortex, 86
Citalopram, 117
Civil War (U.S.), 33
Claviceps purpurea, 190, 191
Coca, 123
Coca-Cola, 123–125
Coca-Cola Company, 125
Coca leaf, 122–123, 125–126
Cocaine, 2, 30, 33, 119, 121–122; effects
    of, 133–138, 140–149, 208; history of,
    122–130; isolation of pure, 125–130
Cocaine psychosis, 129, 138–140, 182
Codeine, 33
Cognition, 183, 211
Coleridge, Samuel Taylor: Kubla Khan, 31
Community mental health movement, 70
Compulsions, 155
Compulsive drug-seeking behavior, 50–51
"Confessions of an English Opium Eater"
    (De Quincey), 30
Congestive heart failure, 29
Consciousness: altered by psychedelic
    drugs, 179, 183, 190, 193, 209–210
Convulsants, 162, 175; selective
    antagonism with sedatives, 174–177
Convulsions, 121, 190
Corpus striatum, 75, 81, 82, 84, 88
Correlation experiments, 74, 77, 82–83,
    118
Cortez, Hernando, 184, 188
Cough medicine(s), 33, 34
Counterculture, 190; see also Hippies
Creese, Ian, 82
Cross-dependence, 165
Cross-tolerance, 164–166
Custance, John, 93
Cyclic AMP (adenosine-3'5'-
    monophosphate), 12, 13, 14, 40, 42,
    81, 82, 83

d-Amphetamine, 134
Da Costa, Jacob, 153–154
Da Costa's syndrome, 153–154
Dahlström, Annica, 142, 199
Deinstitutionalization, 70–71
Delay, Jean, 71–72, 73, 74, 84
Delirium tremens (DT's), 138, 165
Delusions, 114, 139; paranoid, 139, 140;
    in schizophrenia, 62, 87, 209
Dementia praecox, 63
Dendrites, 4–6, 9
Deniker, Pierre, 71–72, 73, 74, 84
Dependence, 32, 40, 121
Depression, 62, 91–93, 132, 152; amine
    hypothesis of, 100, 103, 106–111;
    cocaine in treatment of, 128; diagnostic
    criteria for, 94; drug-induced, 109;
    drugs in treatment of, 2, 98–100, 101,
    113, 117, 208 (see also Antidepressant
    drugs); effect of stimulants on, 121; and
    mania, 93–95, 115, 118;
    norepinephrine and serotonin in, 107,
    109–111; personal accounts of, 92–93;
    stimulants in treatment of, 133–135;
    treatment of, 95–98; types of, 110–111
De Quincey, Thomas, 30–31; "Confessions
    of an English Opium Eater," 30
Diarrhea, 51, 59, 154
"Diet pills," 135; see also Appetite
    suppression
Diethylpropion (Tenuate), 134, 135
Digitalis, 33
Digitalis purpurea, 33
Dimethyltryptamine (DMT), 187, 196, 199
Disease: anxiety as, 151–155; emotional,
    neurological, 16
Distress, free-floating, 155
DOET, 179, 186, 187
DOM (STP), 179, 186, 187
Doors of Perception, The (Huxley), 180–
    181
Dopa, 97
Dopamine, 14, 18, 76, 81, 89, 103, 107,
    109, 140–141, 145; effect of stimulants
    on, 146–149; mapping, 199;
    metabolism of 77–78, 79; in
    Parkinsonism, 74–75; role of, in brain,
    208–209; similarity of psychedelics to,
    195, 196; synthesis of, 141
"Dopamine hypothesis" of schizophrenia,
    148–149
Dopamine pathways, 84–87, 89, 142

Dopamine-receptor sensitivity, 88
Dopamine receptors, 79–83, 86, 87–89,
    208; neuroleptics and, 76–78, 115;
    subtypes, 83, 88
Dosage, 165–166, 211; see also
    Potency(ies)
Dow Chemical Company, 186
Drug abuse, 2, 121, 122, 140, 179;
    amphetamines, 130–33; see also
    Addiction
Drug companies, 16, 41, 72, 130, 159–
    160; development of antidepressants,
    101–103; screening techniques, 139; see
    also Pharmaceutical industry
Drug culture, 132–133, 192
Drug safety, 160–161
Drug therapy, 1, 16, 27, 61, 88, 96, 210;
    in treatment of anxiety, 155, 156–177
Drugs: action mechanism of, 204–205;
    with both therapeutic utility and
    potential for abuse, 121–122, 123–124,
    125, 129–130; dependence-producing,
    29 (see also Addictive potential);
    development of new, 88, 157–159, 177,
    210–211, 212; effects of, 1–3, 14–16,
    140–141, 207–212; illicit, 186; as
    probes, 1, 59, 61, 88–89, 122, 149,
    212; for schizophrenia, 61–89; sculpted
    to fit receptors, 88, 210–211; synthetic,
    131; therapeutic potential of, 23, 34–
    38; understanding of, at molecular
    level, 210, 211; see also Psychedelic
    drugs; Psychoactive drugs; Selectivity of
    action (drugs)

Ego, 155, 205; dissolution of (psychedelic
    drugs), 181; neural basis for
    (hypothesis), 183
Ego boundaries: transcendence of, through
    psychedelic drugs, 181, 183, 193, 205
Eisenhower administration, 70
Electric charge: cell, 6–7; opiate molecules,
    38; peptides, 58, 59
Emotional coloring, 205, 210
Emotional disturbance: in schizophrenia,
    62-63
Emotions, 3, 146; olfaction and, 84–86;
    regulation of, 59, 107, 142, 164, 171,
    207–210, 211; regulation of, by limbic
    system, 47–48, 56, 84

Endorphins, 53–55
Enkephalin derivatives, 57–59
Enkephalins, 18, 53–59, 84, 169, 207, 208, 211
Enlightenment, drug-induced, 179–205
Environment, 95; and schizophrenia, 65, 68
Enzymes, 9, 10, 11, 14, 26
Ephedrine, 131
Epilepsy, 174
Epinephrine, 130–131, 141
Ergocristine, 194
Ergonovine, 191
Ergot, 190–192
Ergot drugs: structures and uses of, 194–195
Ergotamine, 191, 194
Ergotism, 190
Ergotoxine, 191
Ergovine(s), 194
Erlenmeyer, Albrecht, 129
Etorphine, 35
Euphoria, 30, 186; from amphetamines, 131, 132, 133, 135; from cocaine, 128, 129; from heroin, 33, 34, 48; from opiates, 2, 35, 36, 47–48, 50, 84, 95, 208; from stimulants, 121, 148
Evolution, 84, 86, 152
Excitation (cell), 6, 8, 10
Excitation system (brain), 203
Extrapyramidal brain areas, 15–16
Eye: pupils, 47; surgery on, 129–130

Family studies, 65–68, 72, 94–95
Fear: in anxiety, 152–153, 209
Federal Narcotics Hospital, Lexington, Ky., 50
Feeling, 3, 4, 48; effects of opiates on, 42, 43; and thinking, 146
Feeling states: neurotransmitter systems involved in, 207–210
Feelings, 48, 122, 177
Fenfluramine (Pondimin), 134, 136
Ferrosan (drug co.), 168
Fight or flight response, 48, 130, 152
Firing (cell), 7, 8
Firing rate, 8, 12, 36, 81, 149; dopamine neurons, 77, 78, 79; effects of GABA on, 166, 167, 174; in locus coeruleus, 201–203; serotonin-containing neurons, 197–201, 205

Fleischl von Marxow, Ernst, 128–129
Fluoxetine, 117
Folk medicine, 184
Foxglove plant, 33
Franco-Prussian War, 33
Franklin, Benjamin, 114
Freis, Edward, 109
Freud, Sigmund: on anxiety, 154–155; experimental studies on cocaine, 126–129, 130, 133; "On Cocaine," 126–128
Functional phychosis, 138
Fuxe, Kjell, 142, 199

GABA (gamma-aminobutyric acid), 18, 163, 166, 167, 170, 174, 209; binding sites, 175, 176
Gaddum, John, 197
Galen, 29
Garland, Judy, 161
Geigy Drug Company (Basel, Switzerland), 102, 103
Genetic component: in anxiety, 151; in manic-depressive illness, 94–95, 118; in schizophrenia, 68, 72
Genetic predisposition to mental illness, 151
Genetic studies: depression, 91
Giddiness, 153, 154
Glands, 21, 86–87
Glia, 3, 4, 6, 11
Glutamic acid, 19
Glycine, 19
Gonads, 87
Government regulation of drugs, 186, 195
Gram stain, 157
Greengard, Paul, 79–81, 82, 83
GTP (guanosine triphosphate), 12

Haight-Ashbury (San Francisco), 186, 190, 191
Hallucinations, 138, 139, 182; in schizophrenia, 62, 82, 209; in stimulant psychosis, 140
Hallucinogens, 182
Haloperidol, 77, 81, 82, 83, 88
Halsted, William, 129, 130
Headache, 29, 191
Hearing, 180, 205
Heart, 16–19, 22, 36, 105

Heart disease, 29, 33, 153
Heffter, A., 185
Heim, Roger, 189
Hernández, Francisco, 184
Heroin, 2, 29, 33–34, 35, 84, 126; addiction to, 50; euphoria from, 33, 34, 48
Hippies, 132–133, 190, 192
Histamine, 19, 71
Hofmann, Albert, 189–190, 191–193, 196
Homer: Odyssey, 30
Hormonal side effects: neuroleptics, 87, 88
Hormones, 48, 87
Hornykiewicz, Oleh, 75
Hughes, John, 51–53
Human studies: anxiety, 171–173; benzodiazepines, 160, 166
Huxley, Aldous, 181; Doors of Perception, The, 180–181
Hydergine, 191
Hyperactive syndrome, 137–138
Hyper-responsiveness, 203
Hyperventilation, 154
Hypodermic syringe, 33
Hypomania, 93, 94, 114
Hypothalamus, 48, 86
Hypothalamus-pituitary pathway, 87
Hypotheses, scientific, 111, 207

"Idea of reference," 138–139
Imipramine, 98, 101, 102–103, 106, 112
Immunohistochemical techniques, 55
Inca civilization, 123
Information processing, 3, 4, 7, 22
Inhibition (cell), 8, 10
Injection of drugs, 33, 128–129, 132, 133
Insanity, 27, 62, 72
Insecticides, 21–22
Insects, 21
Insomnia, 160, 161
Intestinal contractions: inhibition of, 39, 51–52, 55
Intestinal disturbances, 24, 59
Ion channels, 9–10, 12, 13
Iproniazid, 96–98, 103

Japan: amphetamine abuse in, 132
Johns Hopkins (univ.), 186
Jones, John, 31–32
Journal of the American Medical Association, 131, 132

Kennedy, Edward, 164
Kline, Nathan, 74, 96, 98
Koller, Karl, 130
Kosterlitz, Hans, 51–53
Kraepelin, Emil, 63
Kubla Khan (Coleridge), 31
Kuhar, Michael, 43
Kuhn, Roland, 102–103

Laboratory tools: drugs as, 122; *see also*
    Probes, drugs as
Laborit, Henri, 71
Lactation, 87
Lag-time enigma, 111–112
Lateral geniculate, 145
Leary, Timothy, 193, 195
Librium, 159, 160, 161, 167–169
Lilly Drug Company, 131
Limbic system, 16, 47–48, 84, 86, 88, 142,
    199; benzodiazepine receptors in, 171;
    norepinephrine- and serotonin-
    containing nerve endings in, 107, 146;
    peptide transmitters in, 56; stimulants
    and, 148
Lincoln, Abraham, 114
Linnaeus, Carolus, 24
Lisuride, 201
Lithium, 113–119
Lithium carbonate, 116
Lithium urate, 116
Liver, 50
Locus coeruleus, 48, 141, 145–146, 210;
    effect of psychedelic drugs on, 201–
    202, 203, 204, 205
Loewi, Otto, 16–19, 20
Logan, Joshua, 92
Lophophora williamsii, 184
Lossen, Wilhelm, 126
Low back pain, 157–158
LSD (lysergic acid diethylamide), 2, 132,
    182, 187, 189, 190–195, 196, 203;
    action of, 197, 201; effects of, 179–
    180, 183
LSD psychoses, 193
Lysergic acid, 191

Ma huang (Ephedra vulgaris), 131
Magic mushroom, 188–190
Mania, 61, 93, 112; and depression, 93–
    95, 118; lithium in treatment of, 113–
    119

Manic-depressive illness, 62, 93–95, 138,
    151, 155; incidence of, 94
Mantegazza, Paolo, 123
Mariani, Angelo, 123
Marijuana, 149
Mazindol (Sanorex), 134
MDA, 179
MDMA (Ecstasy), 179, 196, 187, 188
Medications: active principles of, 33
Medicinal drug use, 23, 29, 30, 31, 121–
    122, 123–124, 125, 129–130
Medicine: clinical, 14; folk, 184
Meditation, 183
Memory, 24–25, 36
Mental associations: "loosening" of, 140
Mental function, 25; effect of
    amphetamines on, 135–136;
    biochemistry of, 61; effect of LSD on,
    193; effect of stimulants on, 121, 122;
    higher, 22
Mental hospitals, 68–70
Mental illness: biochemical abnormalities
    in, 72, 151; biologically determined,
    65–68, 94–95; genetic predisposition
    to, 151; psychedelic-drug induced, 182;
    see also under specific illnesses, e.g.,
    Schizophrenia
Mental states: mimicked by psychedelic
    drugs, 183–184
Mephenesin, 158
Meprobamate, 158–159, 160, 161, 165;
    action of, 173–174; binding sites, 175;
    effect on synaptic transmission, 164,
    165, 166; inhibitory effects of GABA
    potentiated by, 166, 174
Merck Drug Company, 126
Mescaline, 2, 187, 190, 197, 199–201,
    203; amphetamine derivative of (TMA),
    186, 188; effects of, 179, 180–181;
    structure of, 196; uses and actions of,
    184–185
Metabolic tolerance, 50
Metabolism, 35, 81; neurotransmitter, 77
Metabolites, 77
Methionine-enkephalin, 56
Methoxyamphetamines, 185–187, 188
Methylphenidate (Ritalin), 134, 135
Methysergide, 203
Methysergide maleate, 195
Mexican Indians, 184–185
Midbrain: periaqueductal gray zone, 47
Miltown. *See* Meprobamate

Minimal brain dysfunction, 137–138
Mitochondria, 9F, 103–104
Mohler, Hans, 167–168
Molecular abnormalities: schizophrenia, 72
Molecular analysis, 59; of antischizophrenic
    drugs, 61, 79
Monoamine oxidase, 14, 96, 97, 99;
    biochemical effects of, 103–104
Monoamine oxidase inhibitors, 96–98,
    101, 102, 103, 106, 109, 117; action
    of, 98–100; side effects of, 100–101
Mood, 2, 14, 112, 122, 208
Mood-altering drugs, 91–119, 121–122
Morpheus (god of dreams), 33
Morphine, 2, 23, 35, 41, 59, 84, 126, 129;
    addiction to, 33, 128–129; brain's own,
    51–59; effect of, 50; three-dimensional
    stucture of, 56; in treatment of pain,
    44
Motivation: anxiety as, 151–152
Motor activity, 15, 75, 84
Muscle-relaxant drugs, 158, 164
Muscle tension, 146
Muscular strength: effect of stimulants on,
    122, 123, 126, 128, 148
Mushrooms, psychoactive, 188–190
Mystical experience, 183–184

Nader, Ralph, 164
Naloxone, 35, 38–39, 41, 51, 52
Narcolepsy, 136–137
National Institute of Drug Abuse, 122
Native American Church of the United
    States, 185
Nature/nurture debate: schizophrenia, 68;
    see also Genetic component
Nepenthe, 30
Nerve activity, 6–7
Nerve-block anesthesia, 130
Nerve ending(s), 4, 7, 8, 9, 55, 99; in
    synaptic transmission, 11, 14
Nervous system: opiate receptors in, 47
Neurasthenia, 133
Neuroleptic drugs, 1, 87–89, 115, 149,
    209, 212; as antischizophrenics, 70–71,
    72–73, 83, 84, 86; clinical effects of,
    78, 79–81, 83, 84, 87–89; clinical
    potencies of, 77, 80, 82–83; discovery
    of, 71–72; and dopamine receptors,
    76–78; impact of, on schizophrenia,
    70–71; as therapeutic agents and as
    probes, 88–89; *see also*

Neuroleptic drugs (*continued*)
 Antischizophrenic drugs
Neurologists, 27
"Neuron doctrine," 8
Neuronal connections, 4–7; discrete/
 branching, 146
Neuronal pathways, 43, 48, 56, 84, 142;
 enkephalin-containing, 55, 57
Neuronal reuptake, 21; *see also* Reuptake
 mechanisms
Neurons, 1, 3–7; discrete, 7, 8;
 organization of, 15; *see also* Firing rate
Neurosciences, 3
Neuroscientists, 2–3
Neurosis, 154–155; anxiety, 153–154
Neurotic depression, 133
Neurotransmission, 59; mechanisms of, 8–
 14
Neurotransmitter inactivation, 103–106
Neurotransmitter mechanisms: aberrant,
 112
Neurotransmitter metabolism, 77
Neurotransmitter receptors, 51, 79, 81,
 82–93; biochemical methods for
 monitoring, 79–81, 84; drug affinity
 for, 88; technique for viewing, 43
Neurotransmitter systems, 208–210, 211–
 212
Neurotransmitters, 8–14, 18–19, 99, 140–
 141; acetylcholine as model, 16–124;
 biogenic amines as, 74; discovery of,
 210, 211; effect of amphetamines on,
 140; effect of drugs on, 14–16; effect
 on mood, 208; effect on neuronal firing
 rate, 149; enkephalins as, 55–56;
 interaction of drugs with, 166–173;
 peptides as, 55–56; studied at
 microscopic level, 84, 212
New England Journal of Medicine, 109
Niemann, Albert, 126
Nigrostriatal pathway, 84
Nomifensine, 117
Nonbenzodiazepine drugs, 173
Norepinephrine, 14, 18, 36, 48, 74, 75, 76,
 77, 82, 103, 109, 140–146, 203, 207;
 effect of iproniazid on, 97; effect of
 lithium on, 118; effect of reserpine on,
 99, 100; effect of stimulants on, 146–
 149; effect on mood, 208; levels of, and
 depression, 105, 106, 107, 109–111;
 mapping, 199; as neurotransmitter,
 103–106; in response to sensory

stimulation, 205; similarity of
 psychedelics to, 195, 196, 201–202;
 structure of, 196; synthesis of, 141
Norepinephrine pathways, 108, 141–142,
 145, 146
Norepinephrine receptors, 111–112
Novocaine, 7
Nucleus accumbens, 84

Obsessional neurosis, 154–155
Obstetrics: use of ergot in, 190, 191
Odyssey, The (Homer), 30
Olfactory tubercle, 84
"On Cocaine" (Freud), 126–128
Ophthalmologic surgery, 129–130
Opiate addiction, 33–34, 48–51
Opiate agonists, 39–42
Opiate antagonists, 35–36, 38, 39–42, 51
Opiate effects, 2; classified by opiate
 receptors, 39–42, 43, 45, 46
Opiate receptors, 29, 40, 51, 52, 53, 55,
 56, 59, 82; and classification of opiate
 effects, 39–42, 43, 45, 46; discovery of,
 167, 168, 207; idealized, 52; location
 of, 42–48
Opiates, 27, 29–59, 84, 168, 212; action
 of, 34–38; death from, 36, 47;
 euphoria produced by, 2, 35, 36, 47–
 48, 50, 84, 95, 208; isolation of active
 ingredient of, 32–33; mixed agonist/
 antagonist, 41–42; in pain relief, 44; as
 therapeutic agents and as probes, 59; in
 treatment of depression, 95
Opium, 2, 29–32, 121, 126; tincture of, 51
Oral administration of drugs, 33, 34, 59
Organic chemistry, 126
Organic psychosis, 138
Osmond, Humphrey, 183
Overdose(s), 35, 160–161

Pahnke, Walter N., 183
Pain: drugs in control of, 1, 29; fast/slow,
 44, 47
Pain impulses, 43–44
Pain perception, 59, 84, 207; brain
 structures in, 43–48
Pain relief, 35, 36, 44, 50, 59
Pain thresholds, 44
Panic: drug-induced, 181–182
Panic attacks, 154, 171
Paranoia, 115

Paranoid schizophrenia, 138–139
Paregoric, 51, 59
Pargyline, 97
Parkinsonian side effects: of
 chlorpromazine, 72, 73, 74; of
 neuroleptics, 72, 73, 74, 75, 76–77, 83,
 84, 88, 115; of reserpine, 73, 74, 75
Parkinson's disease, 72, 75, 78, 84;
 dopamine in, 74–75
Pasternak, Gavril, 39–42, 52
Pemberton, John, 123–124, 125
Penicillin, 50, 157
Peptide neurotransmitters, 55–56, 84, 211
Peptides, 52–55, 211; electrical charge of,
 58, 59
Perception, 15, 16, 177, 211; distorted by
 psychedelic drugs, 179, 182, 183, 209–
 210; disturbances of, in schizophrenia,
 62; *see also* Pain perception; Sensory
 perception
Pert, Candace, 38–42, 43, 51
Peyote, 184–185, 186, 188, 189
Peyotism, 185
Pharmaceutical industry, 98, 100, 210–
 211; and enkephalins, 56–59;
 marketing of lithium, 116–117
Pharmacological analysis, 83
Pharmacologists, 2, 27
Pharmacology, 34, 157
Phendimetrazine (Anorex), 134, 135
Phenmetrazine (Preludin), 134, 135–136
Phenobarbital, 156, 158, 159, 174
Phenothiazine(s), 77
Philip II, king of Spain, 184
Phobias, 155, 156
Phosphoinositide cycle, 14
Pituitary gland, 48, 86, 88
Pituitary hormones, 87
Pizarro, Francisco, 123
Plant extracts, 184; isolation of chemical
 substances from, 126, 189–190
Plants, medicinal, 33
Plath, Sylvia, 93
Plutarch, 91, 93
Poisons, 24
Poppy plant, 29, 30
Postsynaptic neurons, 81, 202
Potassium channels, 9–10
Potency(ies), 35, 174, 204, 211;
 benzodiazepines, 168–169; LSD, 192;
 neuroleptics, 77, 80, 82–83; psychedelic
 drugs, 185–186, 204, 205

Precursor molecules, 8–9, 12, 14
Probes, drugs as, 1, 59, 61, 88–89, 122, 149, 212
Procaine, 130
Prolactin, 87
Promethazine, 71, 77
Prophylactic treatment: depression, 113, 117, 118
Proteins, 38, 53; GTP-binding, 12–14; phosphorylated, 13–14; receptor, 174, 175–176
Psilocin, 187, 190, 196, 199
Psilocybe, 189
Psilocybe mexicana, 189
Psilocybin, 179, 183–184, 187, 196, 199; isolation of, 190
Psychedelic: term, 183
Psychedelic drugs, 2, 27, 149, 179–205; action of, 195–205; classification of, 182–183; effect on sensory stimulation, 203; mental states mimicked by, 183–184; uses and actions of, 184–195; used as probes, 212
Psychedelic experience, 179–183; molecular mechanisms of, 179
Psychiatry: drug therapy in, 1, 16, 27, 61, 88, 96, 210
Psychoactive drugs, 1–3, 7, 27, 149, 207, 209–110; development of, 119; effects of, 121–122, 140–141, 177; therapeutic activity of, 15
Psychoactive plants: isolation of active chemicals of, 189–190
Psychological studies, 73
Psychoses, 62; from cocaine, 129; drug-induced, 179, 181–182, 193; in schizophrenic decompensation, 209; from stimulants, 133, 138–140, 148–149
Psychotherapy, 193; in treatment of anxiety, 153, 155–156
Psychotic depression, 134–135
Psychotic disorders, 93; treatment of, 155
Psychotomimetic effects, 182, 193
Psychotropic drugs, 7
Pyramidal cells, 4

Quinazolines, 159–160
Quinine, 33

Radioassay techniques, 36–39, 52, 82–83, 105

Randall, Lowell, 159–160
Rauwolfia serpentina, 73, 74
Raphe nuclei, 199–201
Receptor-binding techniques, 52, 173–174, 211
Receptor complex, 36
Receptor sensitivity, 112
Receptor sites, 15; opiates, 35, 36–39 (*see also* Opiate receptors); in synaptic transmission, 9, 10, 11–12
Recognition sites, 35, 36, 103, 164–166, 170; GABA, 175; opiates, 82
Recreational use of drugs, 2, 30, 121, 122, 130, 210
Religious ritual: psychedelic drugs in, 184–185, 186, 188–189
Religiousness, 179
Research, 1, 3, 35–36, 43, 59, 61, 84, 212
Reserpine, 14, 73–74, 75, 96–97, 98, 111; action of, 99, 117; as antischizophrenic, 109; biochemical effects of, 104, 109, 112; clinical effects of, 76, 78, 84
Respiration, 47
Reuptake mechanisms, 11, 14, 105–107, 111, 147
Rhone-Poulenc Drug Company, 71
Roche Drug Company (Nutley, N.J.), 159–160, 167
Rockefeller Institute, 191
Roman culture: opium in, 30
Romantics (British), 30
Roosevelt, Theodore, 114

Sadness, 91, 122
San Francisco, 132–133, 186
Sandoz Drug Company, 189, 190, 191, 192, 193
Schizophrenia, 62–64, 93, 94, 140; acute decompensation in, 209; diagnostic criteria for, 64, 65, 66–67, 151; dopamine hypothesis of, 148–149; drug-induced, 139–140, 181–182, 193, 208–209; drugs in treatment of, 1, 96–97 (*see also* Antischizophrenic drugs); incidence of, 65; and incidence of suicide, 96; and society, 61, 65–70; stimulant psychosis and, 138–140; term, 64; treatment of, 115, 155
Schou, Mogens, 116, 117
Scientific discovery(ies), 119; *see also*

Serendipity in science
Scopolamine, 182
Screening techniques, 41, 42, 112, 139, 210–211; benzodiazepine receptors, 173
Second-messenger system, 12–14, 15, 36, 40, 81
Sedation, 1, 156, 157, 159, 164, 166, 171; reserpine-induced, 99; in treatment of mania, 115; tricyclics in, 101
Sedative-convulsant binding sites, 173–177
Sedative-convulsant receptors, 174–177
Sedatives, 72, 160, 161, 173–175; effects of, when mixed with benzodiazepines, 161, 175; selective antagonism with convulsants, 174–177
Seeman, Philip, 82
Seizures, 174
Selective antagonism: sedatives/convulsants, 174–177
Selectivity of action (drugs), 157–159, 164; benzodiazepines, 168, 177, 208, 210, 211–212; and potency, 211
Self-awareness, 186
Senile dementia, 24, 27
Sensation, 205
Sense of self, 181, 183, 203
Sense of space, 181, 183
Sense of time, 180–181, 183
Sensory perception, 43–44, 177; effect of psychedelic drugs on, 179–180, 183, 193, 203
Sensory stimulation, 205; effect on locus coeruleus, 203
Serendipity in science, 96, 119, 159, 210
Serotonin, 18, 74, 75, 76, 82, 103, 109, 207; effect of iproniazid on, 97; effect of lithium on, 118; effect of reserpine on, 99, 100; effect on mood, 208; levels of, and depression, 106, 107, 109–111; similarity of psychedelics to, 190, 195–201; structure of, 196
Serotonin pathways, 198, 199
Serotonin receptors, 112, 197; subtype S$_2$, 205
Sertürner, Friedrich, 33
Shore, Parkhurst, 74
Shulgin, Alexander, 186
Side effects, 115, 211, 212; antidepressants, 111; monoamine oxidase inhibitors, 100–101; nueroleptics, 87, 88; reserpine, 109; *see also* Parkinsonian side effects

Simantov, Rabi, 52, 53
Simon, Eric, 38
Sleeping medications, 156, 158, 160, 161
Smelling behavior, 84–86
Snakeroot plant, 73, 74
Snyder, Solomon H., 38–42, 43, 51, 52, 53
Society: schizophrenia and, 61, 65–70, 71
Sodium, 118
Sodium-binding theory (opiate receptors),
    40–42
Sodium channels, 9–10
Sodium chloride, 39
Sodium ions, 6, 39–42
Somnolence, 50, 208
Somnus (god of sleep), 30
Spaeth, E., 185
Spinal cord, 43–44, 146, 206
Spleen, 105
Squires, Richard, 167–168
Staining techniques, 8, 84, 142–144, 157
Sternbach, Leo, 159–160
Stimulant drugs, 2, 27, 36, 119, 121–149;
    abuse potential, 135; action of, 140–
    149; effects of, 130, 133–138, 208;
    medical uses of, 121–122, 123–124,
    125, 129–130, 133–135, 136–138
Stimulant psychosis, 133, 138–140, 148–
    149
Stoll, Arthur, 190, 191, 192
Stria terminalis, 48
Strychnine, 121
Strychnos nux vomica, 122
Substance P, 18
Substantia gelatinosa, 43, 44
Substantia nigra, 84
Suicide, 2, 96, 109, 111, 160–161, 181,
    193
Sumeria, 30
Surgery, minor, 129–130
Sweden: amphetamine abuse in, 135–136
Sydenham, Thomas, 29
Sympathetic nervous system, 104–106
Symptom(s): anxiety as, 151, 154; in
    anxiety, 152–154, 160; of depression,
    61, 91, 94; of mania, 93; of
    schizophrenia, 62–64, 65, 87, 88
Synapse, 8, 9
Synaptic transmission, 7–14, 27, 97, 103,
    175; effect of benzodiazepines on,

164–166, 174
Synaptic vesicles, 9, 14, 20, 99, 104
Synergistic interactions of drugs, 161, 175
Synesthesia, 180, 183, 203

Tallman, John, 169–170
Tardive dyskinesia, 88, 115
Teonanactl, 188, 189
Terenius, Lars, 38, 52
Terror: in anxiety, 152, 153, 154
Test-tube analysis, 211
Thalamus, 44
Therapeutic agents, 3, 14, 61; development
    of, 16, 27
Theory, scientific, 207; testing of, 111
Therapy: behavioral, 155–156; insight-
    oriented, 186; see also Drug therapy;
    Psychotherapy
Thinking, 3, 4, 16, 22; effect of opiates on,
    42, 43; and feeling, 48, 146; logical,
    15, 145–146
Thought disorder(s), 140; in schizophrenia,
    62–64, 86
3,4,5-Trimethoxyamphetamine (3,4,5-
    TMA), 187
Thyroid gland, 86
Time magazine, 131, 132
TMA, 186
Tolerance, 29, 50, 59, 164–166;
    amphetamines, 132–133;
    benzodiazepines, 160; meprobamates,
    159; opium, 32; stimulants, 133
Tolstoy, Leo, 92
Touch, 205
Touch hallucinations, 140
Tranquilization, 158
Tranquilizing drugs, 1, 27
Transcendental state(s), 183, 203
Tricyclic antidepressants, 14, 100–103,
    105–107, 109, 111, 134–135; action
    of, 117, 147
Tritium, 36, 105
Tryptamines, 187
Tryptophan, 196
Tuberculosis, 96, 98
Twin studies, 65–68, 95
2-Bromo LSD, 197
Tyramine, 100–101

Unconscious, the, 155, 193
Unipolar affective disease, 94–95, 117, 118
Uptake mechanism: norepinephrine, 105,
    106, 107
Uranium, 43
Urea, 115–116
Uric acid, 116
Urine, 115–116
Uterine contractions: ergot-induced, 190,
    191; serotonin-induced, 197

Vagus nerve, 16–19, 20, 24
Valium, 1, 128, 139, 159, 161, 164, 175;
    action of, 167–170; synthesis of, 160
Ventral tegmental area (tegmentum), 84
Vin Mariani (coca extract), 123, 124
Vision, 205; blurred, 154
Visions: drug-induced, 180, 188, 209
Visual hallucinations, 138
Visual perception, 179–180
Visual system, 145–146
Vulnerability, genetic, 95; see also Genetic
    component

Wasson, R. Gordon, 189
Wasson, Valentina, 189
Well-being: drug-induced feelings of, 29,
    30, 133, 208
Western culture: opiate use in, 29–134
Withdrawal: from opium, 32; in
    schizophrenia, 62–63, 73, 87
Withdrawal symptoms, 50; alcohol, 138;
    amphetamines, 137; benzodiazepines,
    160; cross-dependence and, 165;
    meprobamate, 159; stimulants, 133
Wood, Alexander, 33
Woolf, Virginia, 92

Zeller, Albert, 97
Zen (meditation), 183, 184
Zimelidine, 117

Other Books in the Scientific American Library Series

POWERS OF TEN
by Philip and Phylis Morrison and the Office of Charles and Ray Eames

HUMAN DIVERSITY
by Richard Lewontin

THE DISCOVERY OF SUBATOMIC PARTICLES
by Steven Weinberg

THE SCIENCE OF MUSICAL SOUND
by John R. Pierce

FOSSILS AND THE HISTORY OF LIFE
by George Gaylord Simpson

THE SOLAR SYSTEM
by Roman Smoluchowski

ON SIZE AND LIFE
by Thomas A. McMahon and John Tyler Bonner

PERCEPTION
by Irvin Rock

CONSTRUCTING THE UNIVERSE
by David Layzer

THE SECOND LAW
by P. W. Atkins

THE LIVING CELL, VOLUMES I AND II
by Christian de Duve

MATHEMATICS AND OPTIMAL FORM
by Stefan Hildebrandt and Anthony Tromba

FIRE
by John W. Lyons

SUN AND EARTH
by Herbert Friedman

EINSTEIN'S LEGACY
by Julian Schwinger

ISLANDS
by H. William Menard